D1365180

The Effects
of Infant and Child Mortality
on Fertility

Contributors

J. C. BARRETT

YORAM BEN-PORATH

W. BRASS

P. CANTRELLE

LINCOLN C. CHEN

A. K. M. ALAUDDIN
   CHOWDHURY

B. FERRY

DAVID M. HEER

ATIQUR RAHMAN KHAN

JOHN KNODEL

ALAIN LERY

JAMES C. McCANN

POUL C. MATTHIESSEN

VILMA MEDICA

J. MONDOT

SAMUEL H. PRESTON

SHEA RUTSTEIN

JACQUES VALLIN

K. VENKATACHARYA

HSIN-YING WU

The Effects
of Infant and Child Mortality
on Fertility

EDITED BY

Samuel H. Preston

Population Division
United Nations
New York

ACADEMIC PRESS New York San Francisco London
A Subsidiary of Harcourt Brace Jovanovich, Publishers

ACADEMIC PRESS, INC.
111 Fifth Avenue, New York, New York 10003

United Kingdom Edition published by
ACADEMIC PRESS, INC. (LONDON) LTD.
24/28 Oval Road, London NW1

Library of Congress Cataloging in Publication Data

Main entry under title:

The Effects of infant and child mortality on fertility.

   Based on papers from a seminar entitled Infant Mortality in
Relation to the Level of Fertility, held in Bangkok, Thailand, May
6-12, 1975.
   Includes bibliographies.
   1. Fertility, Human—Congresses.   2. Children—
Mortality—Congresses.   3. Infants—Mortality—con-
gresses.   I. Preston, Samuel H.
HB901.E37   301.32′1   77-6608
ISBN 0-12-564440-X

Contents

**Chapter 11 Influence of Variations in Child Mortality
           on Fertility: A Simulation Model Study**   *235*
           K. VENKATACHARYA

List of Contributors

Numbers in parentheses indicate the pages on which the authors' contributions begin.

J. C. BARRETT (209), London School of Hygiene and Tropical Medicine, London, England

YORAM BEN-PORATH (161), The Hebrew University, Jerusalem, Israel and the Maurice Falk Institute for Economic Research in Israel, Jerusalem, Israel

W. BRASS (209), London School of Hygiene and Tropical Medicine, London, England

P. CANTRELLE (181), Office de la Recherche Scientifique et Technique Outre-Mer, Paris, France

LINCOLN C. CHEN (113), Cholera Research Laboratory, Institute of Public Health, Dacca, Bangladesh

A. K. M. ALAUDDIN CHOWDHURY (113), Statistics Branch, Cholera Research Laboratory, Institute of Public Health, Dacca, Bangladesh

B. FERRY (181), Enquête Mondiale de la Fécondité, Office de la Recherche Scientifique et Technique Outre Mer, Yaoundé, Cameroun

DAVID M. HEER (135), Population Research Laboratory, University of Southern California, Los Angeles, California

ATIQUR RAHMAN KHAN (113), National Post Partum Program, Dacca, Bangladesh

JOHN KNODEL (21), Population Studies Center, University of Michigan, Ann Arbor, Michigan

ALAIN LERY (69), Institut National de la Statistique et des Etudes Economiques, Paris, France

JAMES C. McCANN (47), Center for Studies in Demography and Ecology, University of Washington, Seattle, Washington

POUL C. MATTHIESSEN (47), Statistical Institute, Demographic Section, University of Copenhagen, Copenhagen, Denmark

VILMA MEDICA (93), Centro Latinoamericano de Demografia, Santiago, Chile

J. MONDOT (181), Organization for Economic Co-operation and Development, Paris, France

SAMUEL H. PRESTON (1), Population Division, United Nations, New York, N.Y.

SHEA RUTSTEIN (93), Centro Latinoamericano de Demografia, Santiago, Chile

JACQUES VALLIN (69), Institut National d'Etudes Démographiques, Paris, France

K. VENKATACHARYA (235), Department of Statistics, University of Benghazi, Benghazi, Libya

HSIN-YING WU (135), Institute of Public Health, College of Medicine, National Taiwan University, Taipei, Taiwan, Republic of China

CHAPTER 1

Introduction

Samuel H. Preston

This is the first volume to focus on what has become a central concern in modern population studies: the degree to which changes in mortality can be expected to induce changes in fertility. The issue is central because the balance of these forces determines the rate of population growth, which in turn has an enormous array of implications for social welfare. Populations of the twentieth century have enjoyed a mortality decline of unprecedented scope and magnitude. Life expectancy for the world as a whole has grown from less than 30 years of life per birth to more than 50. If a large portion of the mortality decline can be expected to translate routinely into fertility decline, prospects for the future and the case for political intervention would be different from the case where the fertility response is weak. The strength of relations may be an issue in setting levels of mortality-control as well as fertility-control programs. An additional reason for studying these relations is the light they cast on reproductive motivations and behavior themselves.

A variety of possible links between mortality and fertility have long been recognized, but, until recently, careful attempts to identify empirically the strength of any particular relation have been seriously deficient. Authors of demographic transition theory such as Frank Notestein (1945) and Kingsley Davis (1945) suggested that mortality reduction would lead

1

to a fertility reduction because parents would need to bear fewer children in order to achieve a particular desired number of surviving offspring. As Knodel points out in Chapter 2, this notion is at least a century old. In their restatement of demographic transition theory, Coale and Hoover (1958:17) urged caution regarding the strength of the effects, noting that major mortality reductions in Ceylon and Taiwan had not to that point been accompanied by fertility reductions.

Ronald Freedman's massive review of the literature on fertility in 1961 indicated general agreement that a secular decline in mortality must eventually produce a decline in fertility, but he commented that very little systematic empirical work had been done on the subject (1961/62:67). Two years later, in a very influential article, Freedman argued that "known low mortality is one of the necessary conditions for an effective social policy for reducing fertility (1963:164)." Partial evidence for the claim was the statement that, in almost every developed society, a substantial decline in mortality had preceded fertility decline (1963:167). Additional evidence of the importance of the relationships was forthcoming in a cross-national regression analysis by Heer (1966), in which levels of infant mortality were shown to be among the strongest and most consistent predictors of fertility levels.

Useful elaboration of the possible mechanisms relating fertility and mortality occurred during the 1960s. Knodel and van de Walle (1967; Knodel, 1968) emphasized the importance of breastfeeding as an intervening variable linking child mortality with subsequent fertility. Since breastfeeding tends to delay the return of ovulation, the survival of a child should postpone the arrival of the next birth even where no conscious contraception is employed. A second important development was the introduction of survival uncertainty into reproductive models. If parents are concerned with child survival to dates past the end of their reproductive period, then they must anticipate deaths beyond the point where the child could be replaced. If, in addition, the parents are more disturbed by falling short of their "target" number of surviving children than by exceeding it, then the reduced uncertainty resulting from mortality reduction may create a vigorous fertility response. This mechanism was first made operational in a simulation exercise of Heer and Smith (1968), who showed that, in terms of their long-run growth effects, mortality declines could produce a more-than-compensatory fertility decline. These effects were clarified by Schultz (1969), Preston (1972), and O'Hara (1972), but adequate empirical applications of the models were nil.

The early 1970s was a period of almost unguarded optimism about the ability of reductions in child mortality to induce major declines in fertility through preexisting social mechanisms. A distinguished group of demographers was assembled under the auspices of the United States National Academy of Sciences. Their report (1971:87) argued that "policies and programs aimed at reducing infant and child mortality considerably below present levels, therefore, may be an essential underpinning of government programs for fertility control." The United Nations Department of Economic and Social Affairs (1972:84) suggested that "evidence accumulates that the reduction of infant mortality may be a necessary prerequisite to the acceptance of family planning. Couples will not wish to prevent pregnancies until they have some assurance that the children they already have will survive." Most notably, the World Plan of Action adopted at the Bucharest World Population Conference of 1974 contained the following clauses in its section on recommendations for action (United Nations, 1975):

> The short-term effect of mortality reduction on population growth rates is symptomatic of the early development process and must be viewed as beneficial. Sustained reductions in fertility have generally been preceded by reductions in mortality. Although this relationship is complex, mortality reduction may be a prerequisite to a decline in fertility [p. 10];

> While recognizing the diversity of social, cultural, political, and economic conditions among countries and regions, it is nevertheless agreed that the following development goals generally have an effect on the socioeconomic context of reproductive decisions that tends to moderate fertility levels: (a) The reduction of infant and child mortality, particularly by means of improved nutrition, sanitation, maternal and child health care, and maternal education [p. 12].

It is somewhat ironic that the title of the National Academy of Science volume was *Rapid Population Growth* and that the main stimulus for the World Population Conference was concern over the social and economic implications of rapid growth. Such growth had clearly resulted from a failure of fertility declines to match the mortality reduction. But health programs are universally popular and probably do exert an influence on fertility. Since the problem of rapid growth had become redefined exclusively as a problem of high fertility, there seemed to be no inconsistency in simultaneously decrying rapid growth and urging speedier reductions in mortality.

Against this background of hopeful policy declarations resting on a thin research base, the Committee for International Coordination of National

Research in Demography (CICRED) decided to hold a scientific meeting to consider the strength of mortality–fertility relations in different parts of the world. In this matter they received support from the sponsoring agencies of CICRED: the Population Division of the United Nations, the United Nations Fund for Population Activities, and the International Union for the Scientific Study of Population. The seminar was held in Bangkok, May 6–12, 1975, with the added sponsorship of the World Health Organization. Jean Bourgeois-Pichat, Director of CICRED, planned and organized the seminar. Samuel Preston organized the scientific program and commissioned the papers, with the aid of valuable advice from William Brass, Gwendolyn Johnson-Acsadi, and Robert Retherford. Visid Prachuabmoh of Chulalongkorn University was responsible for physical arrangements (see CICRED, 1975).

This volume comprises some of the background papers commissioned for the seminar, revised, edited, and occasionally completely restructured. The comments of Frederick Shorter were instrumental in the revision. An important paper on the subject by Yoram Ben-Porath, which appeared after the seminar's conclusion, has been added. The chapters in this volume are highly focused in order to provide maximum information on the relations of immediate concern. The undoubted influence of fertility on mortality, itself a very worthy topic of investigation, appears here in the guise of a nuisance factor that must be controlled when examining the relations of particular interest. Adult mortality probably influences fertility by affecting the durability of unions and the span of years in which postretirement support will be required. But attention in this volume is focused exclusively on the impact of variation in *child* mortality on fertility. Finally, no detailed consideration is given to the role of health levels, as distinct from mortality, in determining levels of fertility. Health levels almost certainly influence fertility through the probabilities of conception and the length of the reproductive period, and they may have indirect effects through child and adult productivity. Most of these relations involving adult mortality and morbidity would appear to result in a fertility rise when health conditions improve (see Basavarajappa, 1962; Ridley *et al.*, 1967).

The chapters presented here make the largest advance at the level of the individual reproductive couple. The main question addressed is the impact of child death in a family on the parents' subsequent fertility.[1] Although this is not the only level at which effects can emerge, it is certainly

[1] This question had been addressed prior to the Seminar mainly in doctoral dissertations using less than ideal methods. For a brief summary, see Taylor et al. (1976).

the first place to look. However, a couple's own experience with child mortality can also influence the fertility of others through a variety of mechanisms that are discussed later in the chapter.

DEFINING COMPENSATORY RESPONSES IN FERTILITY AT THE FAMILY LEVEL

Under what conditions would fertility's response to variation in child mortality within the family consitute complete compensation in terms of population growth rates? The obvious answer, which is nearly correct, is that complete compensation occurs when the family achieves the same number of surviving children regardless of the number of children who have died. Two qualifications of this conclusion are required. The first is that the same number of surviving children per family will translate into different rates of population growth depending on the average parental age at which the children are born. If higher child mortality requires women to bear additional children when they are older, as seems most likely, then the average age of childbearing will be higher and generations will be stretched out. The same number of surviving children per generation will result in a lower absolute value of population growth on an annual basis. Where growth is positive, higher mortality will result in lower annual growth rates even though the same number of survivors are born per family. This effect is seriously constrained by the social and biological factors that determine the "appropriate" ages of reproduction and is not likely to be quantitatively very important.

A more serious qualification relates to the definition of the phrase, "the same number of surviving children." Surviving to what age? If early infancy, then we are for practical purposes simply talking about the number of births. If we refer to women just at the point where biology ends their reproductive period, then we must consider the survivorship of children to around age 15, on average. Population mathematics eliminates the ambiguity about the appropriate age. In terms of long-run population growth, what counts is the number of offspring who survive to the age of the parents at the time when the children themselves were born. Thus, a completely compensating fertility response achieves the same number of surviving offspring to age 30 or so. When mortality declines, it generally does so at all ages. A fertility strategy that produces the same number of surviving children at the end of reproduction as before the mortality decline will therefore tend to produce more survivors to age 30, and this strategy will not be sufficient to avert an acceleration in population growth when mortality declines.[2]

Both of these qualifications require that a reduction of one child death in the family be matched by a reduction in births of somewhat more than one child in order to leave population growth rates unchanged when mortality levels decline. But it is impractical to deal throughout with generational length and early adult mortality. The chapters in this volume are addressed to the issue of "replacement" rather than that of compensation. Replacement is said to be complete when one additional child death in the family prior to the end of the parents' reproductive life induces one additional birth. The average ratio of additional births to additional deaths is termed *the degree of replacement* or the *replacement rate*. Clearly, complete replacement will generally entail somewhat less than complete compensation.

Some terminological clarity is lost because *replacement* is used in this book not only as a measure but also as a description of a type of behavior. Families in which a child death results in an additional birth are said to have *replaced* the dead child. A replacement *strategy* is one that would

---

[2] The long-run rate of population growth is equal to the intrinsic growth rate (Coale, 1972):

$$r = \frac{\log(NRR)}{T} \cong \frac{\log[p(15)] + \log[_{15}p(30)] + \log(TFR) - \log(1 + SRB)}{T}$$

where

    r = intrinsic rate of natural increase
  NRR = net reproduction rate, or the number of daughters expected to be born to a girl baby who passes through life under the prevailing age-specific mortality and fertility rates
    T = mean length of generation
  $p(15)$ = probability of surviving from birth to age 15
 $_{15}p(30)$ = probability of surviving from age 15 to age 30
  TFR = number of children expected to be born to a girl baby who survives to the end of her reproductive years and is subject at each age to the prevailing age-specific fertility rates
  SRB = sex ratio at birth (males/females)

1. If higher mortality results in a longer length of generation, the intrinsic growth rate will clearly decline in absolute value.
2. If the same number of survivors are produced at the end of reproductive life, then to a close approximation $[\log p(15) + \log(TFR)]$ will be constant. But with lower mortality, $\log [_{15}p(30)]$ will exceed its value when mortality is high. Therefore, r will rise even though compensation for child mortality is complete at the end of reproductive life. The nature of mortality change has been such that, when $p(15)$ rises by 6 units, $_{15}p(30)$ has risen by about 1 unit. Thus, $\frac{1}{7}$ of the growth acceleration that would be produced by mortality decline remains despite pursuit of a strategy resulting in complete compensation at the end of reproduction.

attempt to secure the same number of surviving children at the end of reproduction regardless of the incidence of child death. If the replacement strategy is perfectly successful, then the replacement *measure* will be unity. But it is clear that other mechanisms than a replacement strategy will also affect the measure of replacement. These mechanisms shall now be described in more detail.

MECHANISMS OPERATIVE AT THE FAMILY LEVEL TO AFFECT THE DEGREE OF REPLACEMENT OF DEAD CHILDREN

Interval Effects

Regardless of behavior that may be directed at achieving a certain number of births or surviving children, child death can affect the interval to the next birth. In populations where conscious limitation of family size is negligibly important, the completed family size can be viewed simply as the cumulative outcome of uncorrelated birth intervals spanning a woman's reproductive life. In such populations, it is legitimate to regard intervals and completed family size as simultaneously determined; hence, interval effects translate immediately into fertility effects. In other populations, the importance of interval effects may be lessened by behavior in pursuit of particular goals that produces compensating changes in interval lengths.

The most noteworthy interval effects operate through lactation. Breastfeeding often inhibits ovulation, although the relationship is not deterministic and may vary according to a woman's nutritional level or other characteristics (van Ginneken, 1974; Cantrelle, Ferry, Mondot, Chapter 9). Since breastfeeding would normally be terminated if a nursing child dies, its death may hasten the return of ovulation and consequently speed the arrival of the next birth. More experience with child mortality over the course of a woman's lifetime could be expected to result in more births. This relationship should be most influential in populations where breastfeeding is most common and extended and where nonlactational contraception for spacing purposes is infrequent. The mechanism does not depend on volitional responses of couples to child death, although there is some justification for the view that couples are aware of the contraceptive effects of lactation (Butz and Habicht, 1976: 215). But such recognition is not required for the relation to emerge, and there are undoubtedly many instances where it operates without deliberate choices being made. Other behavior conditioned by the survivorship of a child also falls into the gray

8   Samuel H. Preston

area between conscious choice and passive adherence to biological imperatives and social norms. Indian women who return to their native villages for prolonged periods after childbirth may simply be doing what is expected of them, but they are also practicing abstinence, the most effective form of contraception. In order to identify the effects of these practices, it is unnecessary to know whether their contraceptive value is a recognized or attractive feature of adherence to them.

The amount by which variations in child mortality influence total fertility rates through the interval effects, whether voluntary or involuntary, can be estimated by modifying a model developed by Perrin and Sheps. In this model, the average number of children born in the lifetime of a woman is viewed as the ratio of the length of her reproductive period (in months) to the mean number of months between births. Several components of the mean interbirth interval are recognized: an average waiting time until conception for a woman in the susceptible state, an average period of sterility during pregnancy, and an average period of sterility following the termination of the pregnancy. Infant mortality can be introduced into the model by allowing the sterile period following a live birth to vary according to whether or not the child survives its first year of life. The complete model is

$$TFR = \frac{N}{W + S_0 + IMR(S_1) + (1 - IMR)\ (S_2) + K(W + S_3)}$$

where

N = length of a woman's reproductive life
W = average waiting time until pregnancy for a woman in the susceptible state
S_0 = period of sterility during a pregnancy leading to a live birth
S_1 = period of sterility following a live birth that results in an infant death
S_2 = period of sterility following a live birth that results in a surviving infant
S_3 = period of sterility during and after a pregnancy resulting in a fetal death
IMR = infant mortality rate
K = ratio of chance of a fetal death to chance of a live birth

The sensitivity of fertility with respect to the infant mortality rate may be found by differentiating this latter expression with respect to IMR, a process that yields

$$\frac{dTFR}{TFR} = \frac{(S_2 - S_1)}{I} \cdot dIMR,$$

where I is the average length of the interbirth interval. It can be shown using an expression developed earlier that the intrinsic growth rate would be unchanged if $dTFR/TFR$ were equal to $dIMR$, i. e., if $(S_2 - S_1)/I$ were equal to unity.[3] This latter factor is the difference between the sterile periods associated with a surviving as opposed to a dying infant as a proportion of the entire average interbirth interval. But this factor must be less than unity; it could equal unity only if the dead child could be instantaneously replaced by eliminating the waiting times to conception and the period of pregnancy itself. The interval to the next birth can be shortened by child death, but it cannot be reduced to zero. Hence, replacement cannot be complete, and the growth rate must rise when mortality falls.

Chapters by Cantrelle, Ferry and Mondot and by Chowdhury, Khan, and Chen demonstrate that the interval effects of child death on fertility may be very powerful when breastfeeding is common and extensive. The highest value of $(S_2 - S_1)$ uncovered in this review is 13 months for Bangladesh (Chowdhury, Khan, and Chen). Since a minimum average interbirth interval in a population with extended breastfeeding is surely no less than 26 months, it can be stated with confidence that 50% is the maximum "replacement" response of fertility to changes in infant mortality resulting from this mechanism. That is, it is conceivable that up to half of the increase in growth rates resulting from a reduction in infant mortality could be eliminated by compensating reductions in fertility acting through the interval effects. A more likely level of response in populations with extended breastfeeding is indicated by Potter's analysis of birth intervals in the Punjab. $(S_2 - S_1)$ was 9 months and I was 30 months, a combination that would produce a replacement rate of 30% (Potter et al., 1965:394). Judging from Rutstein and Medica's results, a much smaller response is to be expected in Latin America, where breastfeeding has become much shorter.

Fixed Surviving Children Goals

To the degree that childbearing is goal directed, it is reasonable to suppose that parents bear children not for the rewards accruing from the birth itself but principally for the rewards expected to accrue from surviving children. If the net reward per surviving child declines below zero as

---

[3] According to note 2, the growth rate is unchanged, ceteris paribus, if changes in $\log(TFR)$ and $\log[p(15)]$ are offsetting. Since $dIMR = -d \log[p(15)]$ and $dTFR/TFR = d \log(TFR)$, the two conditions are equivalent.

the number of surviving children increases, then parents should set some sort of numerical target for surviving children. If the rewards continue to be positive throughout the achievable range, then the appropriate strategy is simply to take "as many as God sends."

Presuming that a target number of surviving children is set within the achievable range but not at its extremes, then considerations of child mortality should influence fertility. Two different strategies can be distinguished, although in practice they may coexist for a particular couple.

Replacement Strategy

Parents intend to have x children alive at the end of their reproductive period. They first attempt to bear x children. If any die before the end of reproduction, they attempt to have a replacement birth. If one of the replacement births dies, they attempt to replace it. They practice contraception whenever they have x living children within the reproductive period.

Insurance (Hoarding) Strategy

Parents intend to have x children alive at some point in the future. They are aware that some of their children may die before that point but beyond the stage where they are physiologically able to replace them. Therefore they attempt to bear more than x children even if none die as a form of insurance against subsequent deaths. They practice contraception only when they are "reasonably" sure that the target will be achieved or when falling short is in some sense less costly than exceeding it.

These are obviously simplifications of what could be exceedingly complex "inventory control" problems. But it is probably reasonable to apply no more sophisticated reasoning to the problem than parents themselves would. The key distinction is between a passive, adaptive strategy of replacement and an active, anticipatory strategy of insurance. In the former case, the magnitude of effects can be readily estimated from family-level reproductive and survival histories. In the latter case, it is important to know what parents are thinking and what their perceptions of expected child mortality are. To the degree that expectations of future child mortality are based on child mortality experience within the family, the consequences of insurance strategies can be studied through exactly the same designs used in the study of replacement strategies. If they are partially framed on the basis of the experience of others with child mortality, then a complete design should include that experience as a variable.

The operation of insurance strategies in which nonfamilial experience informs a family's own expectations poses serious design problems for studies focusing on the individual couple. The chapter by Heer and Wu is the most careful attempt yet made to come to grips with these problems. However, there are reasons to believe that for the most part a "pure" insurance strategy is less efficient than a "pure" replacement strategy, and hence that most couples will emphasize the latter. Because the large majority of child deaths will occur prior to even a very late target age, they can be observed and reacted to during the reproductive period itself and need not be anticipated. By the end of the parents' childbearing period, their children will be on average 10 to 15 years old. Very few will have to pass through the most hazardous first two years of life. Parents must anticipate child survival not through the entire age span to adulthood but in fact through what tend to be the ages of lowest mortality. For example, if 10 children are born at two-year intervals to women starting at age 20 in a population with life expectancy of 35, then 74.5% of the deaths those children will experience prior to age 30 will have occurred prior to the mother's attainment of age 40; at a life expectancy of 60, the figure is 68.3% (compiled from Coale and Demeny, 1966:8, 18).

The relative importance of replacement versus insurance strategies will depend on the age to which parents target the survival of their children. The higher that age, the more insurance strategies should dominate replacement ones. Countries where the primary functions of offspring are support for parents in their older years, perpetuation of the family line through their own offspring, performance of ceremonial burial activities, etc., should show stronger relative insurance effects at the same level of mortality than countries where parents are more interested in children qua children.

The timing of the different mechanisms will probably differ substantially. When mortality levels decline, interval effects should be nearly fully realized within a time period equal to the average interbirth interval; effects of replacement strategies must be achieved within a period equal to the length of women's reproductive years; effects through insurance strategies may take much longer to work themselves out, because they require that mortality changes be perceived and incorporated into expectations.

REASONS WHY REPLACEMENT MAY BE INCOMPLETE

The principal conclusion of this volume is that, on average, an additional child death in the family, ceteris paribus, leads to far less than one additional birth. The interval effects are reasonably strong in the high fertility, extensively breastfeeding populations of Bangladesh and tropical Africa. But as we have indicated such effects cannot begin to produce complete replacement. Behavior consistent with replacement or insurance strategies is far more difficult to detect. The chapters by Rutstein and Medica, Chowdhury and Khan and Chen, and Knodel indicate that such strategies are virtually inoperative in the high fertility, essentially pretransitional populations they review. In order to draw such conclusions, it is necessary to remove interval effects from the calculations; both Knodel and Chowdhury, Khan, and Chen independently develop a procedure for doing so.[4]

On the other hand, the chapters by Heer and Wu, Vallin and Lery, Knodel, and Ben-Porath suggest that a replacement strategy is clearly evident in populations farther along on the transitional scale. But in no population are as many as 50% of child deaths replaced by additional births, once proper statistical controls are instituted. It is important to recognize that many statistical pitfalls—many of them unavoidable in the data sets exploited—reduce the reliability of measured effects. As documented in the chapter by Brass and Barrett, most of these would tend to produce an upward bias in the measured effect of mortality on fertility. An important effect operating in the opposite direction is memory error regarding events and dates of births and child deaths.

The methods used in these chapters fall into two main classes: analysis of stopping probabilities or their complement, parity progression ratios (Vallin and Lery, and Ben-Porath), and examination of cumulative fertility behavior subsequent to child death versus child survival (Heer and Wu, and Knodel). The comparative experience in cumulative fertility has a straightforward interpretation. The logic underlying the use of stopping probabilities is the following. Some fraction of women achieving a particular parity (number of live births) plan to stop childbearing at that point, providing that their last child survives. This fraction, S, may be inferred by observing the fraction of women whose last child survives who do in fact stop. The death of the last child induces a certain additional fraction of women so affected to continue on to the next parity, given a total fraction who stop in this category of S'. The fraction, $(S - S')/S$, is thus interpretable as the proportion of women who would have stopped childbearing but who are induced to continue as a result of child death. This reasoning can be applied to all children as well as to last children. The results of Lery and Vallin's analysis of French women suggests that replacement is about one-third complete on this measure, and Ben-

---

[4] The procedure was also used in Adlakha (1973) with different results. Adlakha finds that the average extension of the interbirth interval produced by child survival is longer than that which could plausibly be attributed to breastfeeding and that child deaths of birth order n tend to shorten the length of interval between orders $n + 1$ and $n + 2$. His sample is based on 803 married women in Ankara.

Porath's results suggest a replacement rate of about one-sixth among Israeli women (Table 8.3). Ben-Porath further shows that the death of a child affects the probability of stopping at the *next* parity by about the same order of magnitude, but effects are negligible beyond that point.

There are many reasons why replacement might be incomplete, and the results presented in this volume cannot distinguish effectively among them. But it is worthwhile to list some of the major possibilities:

1. If there is no target number of surviving children. Childbearing behavior may be totally responsive to nonnumerical considerations, e.g., sexual gratification or fulfillment of social or religious expectations regarding marriage, pregnancy, and the appropriate behavior for a fecund woman.

2. If the target number is so high that it could not be achieved even if all children survived. Obviously child survival will not condition fertility in this case.

3. If family size targets are framed for one sex only. The death of a child of the other sex would induce no fertility response; death or survival of that sex is basically immaterial. It is not the case that the dead child of the unwanted sex is not "replaced"; either the dead or the surviving child must be replaced by a child of the desired sex. This type of behavior is simulated in the chapter by Venkatacharya, who demonstrates the marked acceleration of population growth that accompanies mortality decline when parents pursue a replacement strategy aimed at one sex only. The results of this chapter stand in marked contrast to the earlier effort by Heer and Smith to simulate an insurance strategy. Completely asymmetric sex preferences are not required; any behavior in pursuit of a particular sex composition of children would lead to a similar attenuation of the replacement effect.

4. If control over fertility is imperfect. Those experiencing a child death may be unable to replace it because of fecundity impairments, death or absence of a husband, or fetal loss. On the other hand, those not experiencing a child death and achieving their target may be unable to prevent the birth of another child who would constitute a replacement birth for another woman. These excess births would reduce the measured impact of child mortality on fertility. Furthermore, if the unwanted child died, no attempt would be made to replace it. The evidence in the chapter by Heer and Wu that the desire for additional children is more responsive to child mortality than are actual births is a good indication that imperfect fertility control may be fundamentally important in explaining the incompleteness of replacement. Evidence on the use of contraception in Rutstein and Medica and in Heer and Wu bears additionally on this point.

5. If the child death produces a downward modification of the reproductive target. Many possibilities may be suggested. The unpleasant experience of offspring mortality may make couples recoil from the prospect of exposing themselves again to the risk. From the purely economic standpoint, a child death may raise the perceived costs of raising a surviving child and thus produce a substitution effect away from expenditure on children. Ben-Porath also suggests that a family's wealth position is compromised by child death and that a negative wealth effect on reproductive targets may ensue.

6. If the child death had been anticipated in advance and protected against by an insurance strategy. Two possibilities must be distinguished here. One occurs when the expectation of future child mortality used as a parameter in selecting the number of insurance births is based completely upon familial experience. In this case, the observed degree of replacement in the family will be an accurate indicator of child mortality effects, although behavior will depend on the birth order of the child in a different fashion than it would under a strict replacement strategy (stronger reaction to low birth order deaths, weaker to higher birth order deaths). In the other case, expected child mortality is at least partially based on experience outside the family. To repeat, the extrafamilial effects of mortality cannot be captured within the analytic strategies pursued for the most part in this volume. If these are powerful because insurance strategies predicated on extrafamilial experience are prevalent, then replacement effects will understate the consequences of mortality decline for fertility reduction. We have tried to argue that this is probably not a fundamentally important qualification, and Heer and Wu's demonstration that perceptions of child survival risks are essentially unrelated to fertility provides some empirical support for the claim. On the other hand, they also demonstrate that such perceptions were not reliably measured and that the community mortality level did exert a significant impact on fertility apart from familial experience. However, they also note that the community mortality level may be a proxy for a whole list of development indicators and thus cannot be unambiguously interpreted.

These obstacles to replacement are undoubtedly present in every population, with varying distributions of women among the categories. The obstacles are clearly expected to be greatest in populations with high average family size goals, fatalistic attitudes toward reproduction, son preference, high secondary sterility, and poor contraceptive technology. It is therefore not surprising to find the least evidence of replacement strategies among populations at low levels of social development. On the other hand, the replacement rate receives a significant boost from interval effects in such populations. What is more surprising is that these obstacles in the aggregate are sufficiently large in every population reviewed that only a small fraction of mortality variation at the family level seems to translate into fertility variation. The picture is not attractive for those who look to mortality reduction as a means of reducing fertility through familial effects, let alone for those who advocate such measures as a means to reduce growth rates. Nor does it lend much support to models of fertility decision making that view couples as proceeding deliberately and with minimal encumbrances toward some target number of surviving children.

EXTRAFAMILIAL EFFECTS OF CHILD MORTALITY ON FERTILITY

For the most part, the results in this volume do not bear on extrafamilial mortality influences on couple fertility behavior. In addition to insurance effects predicated on group mortality levels, many such influences need to be considered in a complete analysis of the consequences of mortality change. One of the most plausible modes of influence operates through marriage systems. In preindustrial Europe, the evolution and diffusion of the societal norm that a husband should himself be directly responsible for the support of his wife and children, combined with an agrarian mode of production in which the resources for such support—primarily land— were strictly limited in the aggregate, provided the possibilities for major responses of fertility to mortality change. A mortality crisis would increase the number of new widows and widowers, heirs and heiresses, and increase the chances of marriage and parenthood for single people who survived (see Eversley, 1957 for a vivid example of the expected marriage and fertility response to an episode of very high mortality). No couple, of course, need be aware that mortality conditions had changed for the fertility response to be forthcoming. The same type of mechanism would operate where accumulation of a fixed bride price or dowry was a prerequisite to marriage; population pressure at the family level caused by mortality decline would serve to delay the marriage of offspring:

Fertility change is only one possible response to a mortality change, and whether it is activated undoubtedly depends upon many conditioning factors in the society. Geertz (1968) demonstrates with evidence from Java that fertility cannot be expected to respond to mortality change where land is allotted at the village level on the basis of family "need." Friedlander (1969) points out that even where the European marriage pattern was in effect, the relation between societal levels of fertility and mortality was attenuated where "safety valves" for population pressure exist. He suggests that the long lag between mortality and fertility declines in England is plausibly attributed to the simultaneous occurrence of industrialization and its rural–urban migration possibilities. Overseas migration, geographic extension of the resource base, and labor intensification of agriculture may, under the right circumstances, also offer safety valves. Some of these alternative responses can themselves indirectly affect fertility. For example, net rural–urban migration exposes increasing proportions of the population to what is conventionally a lower fertility context. In all cases, it appears that mortality declines may reduce fertility through extrafamilial mechanisms only by introducing a stage of chronic deprivation in the form of sexual abstinence, forced migration, declining standards of living, or sacrifice of leisure. Policymakers could find little comfort in such mechanisms even if they could be shown to be powerful.

The complexity of the societal-level relationships is reflected in the chapter by Matthiessen and McCann. Both cross-regional and longitudinal relations between mortality and fertility in Europe are highly varied and provide support for few empirical generalizations, although the time-series picture is somewhat clarified when attention is extended to child as well as to infant mortality. This diversity of results is somewhat surprising since fertility levels undoubtedly exert a positive influence on mortality levels in most situations and since both mortality and fertility should respond independently but in the same direction to socioeconomic modernization. These contaminating influences should help to create the appearance of a positive relation at the aggregate level, although variation in morbidity from diseases, such as malaria, that affect reproductive performance operates in the other direction (as shown by Cantrelle, Ferry, and Mondot). Brass and Barrett emphasize that the difficulties of implementing an effective research design for studying relations at the aggregate level are much more severe than the difficulties of analyses conducted at the individual level. Continued pursuit of the aggregate relations is probably the most important business left unfinished in this collection, and Brass and Barrett point the way toward some methodology that would be usefully applied. The final word on effects at the family level has not been written, but the results presented here are sufficiently consistent and plausible that few surprises should be expected when it is.

One final extrafamilial response to mortality change should be mentioned. Powerful formal governmental structures now exist to convert social distress signals into policy. The repertoire of reactions to mortality change need no longer be circumscribed by longstanding informal norms, customs, and institutions. In a very real sense, the tremendous volume of international financial and human resources now being directed toward "the population problem" is a social response to mortality decline. This response is surely as variable as any, but in view of the apparent inadequacy of apolitical mechanisms for reestablishing zero growth, it is reassuring that more powerful devices exist and are beginning to be exploited.

REFERENCES

Adlakha, Arjun
  1973   "Fertility and mortality: An analysis of Turkish data." Demography India Volume II(1).
Basavarajappa, K. G.
  1962   "Effect of declines in mortality on the birth rate and related measures." Population Studies Volume 16(1), 237–56.
Butz, William P. and Habicht, Jean-Pierre
  1976   "The Effects of Nutrition and Health on Fertility: Hypotheses, Evidence, and Interventions." Pp. 210–38 in Ronald Ridker, (ed.), Population and Development: The Search for Selective Interventions. Baltimore: Johns Hopkins Press.
CICRED
  1975   Seminar on Infant Mortality in Relation to the Level of Fertility, 6–12 May, 1975. Bangkok, Thailand. (Articles in original language; Introduction and Conclusion in English, French, and Spanish.)
Coale, Ansley J. and Edgar M. Hoover
  1958   Population Growth and Economic Development in Low-Income Countries. New Jersey: Princeton University Press.
Coale, Ansley J. and Paul Demeny
  1966   Regional Model Life Tables and Stable Populations. New Jersey: Princeton University Press.
Davis, Kingsley
  1945   "The world demographic transition." Annals of the American Academy of Political and Social Science 237:1–11.
Eversley, D. E. C.
  1957   "A survey of population in an area of Worcestershire from 1660 to 1850 on the basis of parish registers." Population Studies 10:253–79.
Freedman, Ronald
  1961/62   "The sociology of human fertility: A trend report and bibliography. Current Sociology 10–11(2):35–119.
  1963   "Norms for family size in underdeveloped areas." Proceedings of the Royal Society B 159:220–45.
Friedlander, Dov
  1969   "Demographic responses and population change." Demography 6(4):359–82.
Geertz, Clifford
  1968   Agriculture Involution. University of California Press, Berkeley.
Heer, David M.
  1966   "Economic development and fertility." Demography 3(2):423–44.
Heer, David M. and Dean O. Smith
  1968   "Mortality level, desired family size, and population increase." Demography 5(1):104–21.
Knodel John
  1968   "Infant mortality and fertility in three Bavarian villages: An analysis of family histories from the 19th century." Population Studies 22:297–318.

Knodel John and E. van de Walle
  1967 "Breastfeeding, fertility, and infant mortality: An analysis of some early German data." Population Studies 21:109–131.
National Academy of Sciences
  1971 Rapid Population Growth: Consequences and Policy Implications. Baltimore: Johns Hopkins Press.
Notestein, Frank W.
  1945 "Population—the long view." Pp. 36–57 in Theodore W. Schultz, (ed.), Food for the World. Chicago: University of Chicago Press.
O'Hara, Donald J.
  1972 "Mortality risks, sequential decisions on births, and population growth." Demography 9(3):485–98.
Potter, Robert G., Mary L. New, John B. Wyon and John E. Gordon
  1965 "Application of field studies to research on the physiology of human reproduction: Lactation and its effects upon birth intervals in eleven Punjab villages, India." Pp. 377–99 in Mindel C. Sheps and Jeanne C. Ridley (eds.), Public Health and Population Change. Pittsburgh: University of Pittsburgh Press.
Preston, Samuel H.
  1972 "Interrelations between death rates and birth rates." Theoretical Population Biology 3(2):162–85.
Ridley, Jeanne Clare, Mendel C. Sheps, Joan W. Lingner and Jane A. Menken
  1967 "The effects of changing mortality on natality: Some estimates from a simulation model." Milbank Memorial Fund Quarterly 45(1):77–97.
Schultz, T. Paul
  1969 "An economic model of family planning and fertility." Journal of Political Economy 77(2):153–80.
Taylor, Carl, J. S. Newman and Narindar U. Kelley
  1976 "The child survival hypothesis." Population Studies 30(2):263–78.
United Nations, Department of Economic and Social Affairs
  1972 Measures, Policies, and Programs Affecting Fertility, with Particular Reference to National Family Planning Programs. Population Study No. 51, New York.
United Nations
  1975 Report of the United Nations World Population Conference, 1974. Bucharest, August 19–30, 1974. E/CONF. 60/19. New York.
van Ginneken, Jeroen K.
  1974 "Prolonged breastfeeding as a birth spacing method." Studies in Family Planning 5:201–06.

Part 1

THE EUROPEAN RECORD

CHAPTER 2

European Populations in the Past: Family-Level Relations

John Knodel

One of the most prominent issues in the early literature on the decline of fertility in European countries concerned the relationship between declining child mortality and falling fertility rates. The issue gained salience after the formulation of the demographic transition model which attributes central importance to the timing and interdependence of the secular declines in birth and death rates in Western demographic experience. Actually, even in preindustrial times some attention was given to the relationship between levels of fertility and child mortality. In the German literature as early as 1861, before fertility showed any sign of declining, Wappäus posited the following connections:

> First of all, a mother whose child was stillborn or died soon after birth generally gives birth sooner to another than a mother who nurses and rears her live born child. Second, as a rule it can be assumed that each parental couple wishes to raise a certain number of children and therefore when they already have this number of living children they no longer so actively want to enlarge the family as when the desired number has not been reached due to the loss of infants shortly after birth [Wappäus, 1861: 322].

Wappäus states the two main ways the child mortality experience of individual couples might affect their fertility. The first, which has been labeled the *physiological effect,* relates the average length of a birth interval to the fate of the infant born at the onset of the interval in circumstances where mothers typically nurse newborn children. There is ample evidence that lactation inhibits conception through prolonging postpartum amenorrhea (see, e.g., Van Ginneken, 1974). The death of an infant, by prematurely interrupting lactation, allows ovulation to be resumed sooner and, in the absence of contraception, results in an earlier subsequent pregnancy. The second, labeled the *child replacement effect,* implies that couples continue to produce children, replacing those who die young, until they reach some number of surviving progeny they consider sufficient. Implicit in the operation of this second effect is the assumption that couples are able to practice some means of family limitation once the desired number of children is attained.

   Both effects, if they operate, should be apparent in the reproductive histories of individual couples, since the influence being exerted on fertility behavior arises from the couple's own direct experience with child mortality. The purpose of the present chapter is to review the evidence on the extent of these two effects in European populations in the past, based on individual data. Other influences of child mortality on fertility have been suggested, but they cannot be adequately examined with individual-level data. These include a mechanism whereby couples adjust their fertility to anticipate possible future child deaths, thus insuring the survival of at least the minimum number of offspring considered sufficient (Heer and Smith, 1968). This "insurance" effect assumes that couples have some awareness of the community level of child mortality independent of their own experience and adjust their fertility with these risks in mind. Finally, we can mention a societal effect which would operate indirectly through social customs to insure that the community's fertility level was brought into some sort of balance with the community level of general mortality (including child mortality). Such customs might govern age of marriage or breastfeeding practices in ways totally independent of an individual couple's fertility intentions. Indeed, there need be no general recognition among the population of the connection between these social customs and their consequences.

   It is worth noting at the start that the relationship between mortality and fertility is complicated by a multitude of additional influences acting on each of the main variables and that this relationship can be self-reinforcing with the influences operating in both directions. It is therefore particularly difficult to isolate the direct influence of infant mortality on fertility in such a manner that interpretation becomes unambiguous.

   The use of individual family histories to study demographic behavior in the past is a relatively recent development. In the last two decades, however, family reconstitution (i.e., linking together the entries of births, marriages, and deaths from parish records or similar sources into family histories of vital events) has become a central technique to historical demography, and the number of studies analyzing reconstituted family data has proliferated. Examination of the effect of an infant death on the length of the subsequent birth interval, i.e., the physiological effect of infant mortality on fertility, is routinely reported in many of these studies. Unfortunately, with few exceptions (e.g., Knodel, 1968, 1970; Smith, 1972), little attempt has been made to examine other possible effects of child mortality on fertility. Part of the reason for this is probably that many of the studies deal with populations during preindustrial periods when fertility was high and apparently uncontrolled by deliberate attempts at family limitation. Under these circumstances, it may have been assumed that only the physiological effect of infant mortality on fertility was operating. Even in the studies that show clear evidence of the onset of family limitation, however, no attempts were made to examine changes in the relationship between these two important variables. Fortunately, several of the monographs based on reconstituted family data include appendix tables of basic data which permit at least some further analysis of the influence of infant mortality on fertility.

Most of the results presented in the remainder of the paper refer to periods prior to the secular decline in marital fertility associated with the demographic transition. Although special attention will be focused on the few situations where there is clear evidence of the onset of fertility reduction during the period covered, the relationship of child mortality and fertility during the predecline period is also of interest. One of the more striking findings of a study utilizing aggregate level data for nineteenth-century Germany was the strong positive correlation between levels of infant mortality and marital fertility in Bavarian districts where breastfeeding was customarily uncommon at a time when fertility had yet to start on the path of secular decline (Knodel and van de Walle, 1967). Furthermore, the same study showed that in a large number of German areas for which data on breastfeeding customs were available, strong positive correlations between infant mortality and marital fertility persisted even after differences in breastfeeding were statistically controlled. Such findings raise the question of whether a comparable relationship between infant mortality and fertility existed on the individual level independent of the physiological effect.

INFANT MORTALITY AND BIRTH INTERVALS

In situations in which deliberate attempts to control fertility are absent (i.e., natural fertility prevails) and in which women typically breastfeed their children for extended periods of time, the physiological effect of infant mortality on fertility should be apparent in a comparison of birth intervals following infant deaths with normal birth intervals, i.e., those in which the child born at the onset survives infancy. Table 2.1 summarizes the results of a number of studies which make this comparison for European populations during periods of assumed natural fertility. It should be noted that natural fertility does not necessarily imply that fertility is at its biological maximum but rather that no deliberate actions are taken by couples to stop childbearing once a given family size is achieved. Natural fertility is virtually always kept below its biological maximum by social custons—such as those governing breastfeeding or seasonal migration separating spouses—which operate independently of the number of children already born (Henry, 1961).

   In only three of these areas, the German villages of Mömmlingen, Anhausen, and Schönberg, was direct evidence on breastfeeding customs available. According to a survey conducted at the turn of this century, as well as other supporting evidence, Mömmlingen is located in an area where almost all mothers were known to breastfeed their children for extended periods while Schönberg and Anhausen are situated in areas where any breastfeeding at all was uncommon and extended breastfeeding (over 6 months) virtually nonexistent (Knodel, 1968). It is therefore of particular interest to observe that the smallest average differences between normal intervals and intervals following infant deaths characterize the two villages where breastfeeding was known to be uncommon (and hence would hardly operate as the link between infant mortality and the length of the birth interval) and that the village where extended breastfeeding was known to be common is characterized by one of the largest differences. From our limited knowledge of breastfeeding customs in Europe, it appears that during the late nineteenth century at least, mothers avoided nursing infants in wide areas of central Europe, including southern Baden, Württenberg, and Bavaria as well as parts of Austria, Bohemia, and Saxony (Knodel and van de Walle, 1968). Although equivalent information may be lacking for many other parts of Europe, it is at least worth noting that the other villages shown in Table 2.1 do not fall in these areas where extended breastfeeding was known to be uncommon. The average duration of birth intervals following infant deaths, and therefore minimally influenced by the prevailing breastfeeding customs, clusters in a narrow range of about 19 to 22 months with only a few exceptions.

   The evidence in Table 2.1 suggests forcefully that the physiological effect of infant mortality on fertility was operating in preindustrial European populations, except in those areas where breastfeeding was uncommon. Several related questions, however, merit answering: *(a)* Do studies

TABLE 2.1

Intervals between Successive Confinements According to the Fate of the Infant Born at the Beginning of the Interval: Results from Studies of Periods of Assumed Natural Fertility

Village or group	Country	Year of marriage	Mean interval (months)		Difference in mean intervals
			After infant survival	After infant death	
Saint Patrice	France	1640–1780	29.4	16.5	12.9
Mömmlingen	Germany	1840–1890	30.0	19.4	10.6
Bilheres-d'Ossau	France	1740–1790	32.3	21.7	10.6
Glostrup	Denmark	1677–1790	30.7	20.3	10.4
Troarn	France	1660–1760	30.6	20.8	9.8
Tourouvre-au-Perche	France	1665–1765	30.0	20.7	9.3
Crulai	France	1674–1742	29.6	20.7	8.9
Geneva bourgeoisie	Switzerland	Before 1650[a]	29.5	22.1	7.4
Rumont	France	1720–1790	27.8	20.7	7.1
Sachsen Miners	Germany	Before 1880	26.9	20.5	6.4
Thézels-St. Semin	France	1700–1792	31.9	26.1	5.8
Ile-de-France villages	France	1740–1780	27.2	21.4	5.8
French Canadians	Canada	1700–1729	25.0	19.4	5.6
Scotteville-les-Rouen	France	1760–1790	24.1	19.3	4.8
Bléré	France	1707–1765	22.8	18.6	4.2
Meulan	France	1660–1739	26.1	22.4	3.7
Tonnerrois parishes	France	18th century	23.8	21.6	2.2
Schönberg	Germany	1840–1890	22.0	20.0	2.0
Anhausen	Germany	1840–1890	19.9	19.7	0.2

Sources: Anhausen, Mömmlingen, and Schönberg from Knodel (1968); Bléré calculated from data given in Lachiver (1969a); Crulai from Gautier and Henry (1958); French Canadians from Henripin (1954); Meulan from Lachiver (1969b); Rumont calculated from Robert (1969); Sachsen Miners from Giessler (1885); all others from Smith (1974).

[a] Birth years of husbands.

of the effect of breastfeeding on postpartum sterility yield results which would indicate that the physiological effect of infant mortality on fertility could alone account for differences in birth intervals of the magnitude found in the studies of preindustrial populations just reviewed? *(b)* How much of a reduction in fertility could we expect from the physiological effect of infant mortality alone if a major reduction in infant mortality took place? *(c)* Is there any internal evidence in the family history data to indicate that infant mortality affects the length of birth intervals in a manner independent of the physiological effect? The rest of this section attempts to answer each of these questions in turn.

Essentially, all studies utilizing direct evidence on lactation and either postpartum amenorrhea or postpartum resumption of ovulation indicate that breastfeeding extends postpartum sterility. The extent of this effect, however, varies substantially from study to study. For example, Salber and her colleagues found a difference of only 4 months in the median duration of amenorrhea between mothers in the Boston area who did not breastfeed their children at all and those who breastfed for almost a year (Salber *et al.*, 1966). A number of studies based on women in less developed countries indicate that lactation extends the average duration of amenorrhea up to 9 or 10 months (e.g., Potter *et al.*, 1965; Van Ginneken, 1974), and recent data from a small sample in Bangladesh revealed a median period of 17 months of amenorrhea for women with surviving breastfed children in comparison to a period of only 2 months for women whose infants died neonatally (Chen *et al.*, 1974). It appears that the physiological effect of lactation on fertility is itself subject to other influences such as the intensity of breastfeeding and nutritional differences (Potter, 1975). There is evidence that partial breastfeeding (i.e., done in conjunction with supplementary feeding) is less effective in suppressing ovulation than full breastfeeding (Van Ginneken, 1974). Other research has also indicated that lactation extends amenorrhea longer among poorly nourished women (Frisch, 1974). The important point for the present discussion is that it is not possible to determine how much influence lactation alone exerts on fecundability in a particular population without taking into account the other factors that affect this relationship. In preindustrial Europe, the nutritional level was probably not especially good among the rural peasantry or working classes, and thus we might expect the impact of lactation on amenorrhea to be closer to the maximum than the minimum. Of course, not all infants who die before age 1 die immediately after birth, so that a mother who loses an infant may have nursed it for a number of months. Typically, in preindustrial European populations, over 40% of infant deaths occurred within the first month of life (Wrigley, 1968) so that the average age of death of infants dying before their first birthdays is closer to 3 months than half a year. Since the effect of the first couple of months of lactation on postpartum sterility tends to be minimal (probably because even in the absence of lactation women typically experience several months of anovulatory cycles), average differences of up to 8 or 9 months between normal birth intervals and birth intervals following infant deaths can plausibly be accounted for by the physiological effect alone. Even larger differences might be attributable solely to this effect, but—with the exception of the study from Bangladesh mentioned earlier—they would exceed the range of differences found in most studies on modern populations that observe the physiological impact of lactation directly.

Even assuming that the physiological effect of infant death could reduce the average birth interval by as much as 10 months, a substantial reduction in infant mortality would yield only a small reduction in fertility as a result of this mechanism alone. The magnitude of this effect can be estimated fairly easily. Assume that two cohorts of women marry at the same age and cease childbearing at the same age. Suppose that for one cohort 25% of children died before age 1 ($_1q_0$ = .25), a level as high as or higher than that experienced by most of the populations covered in Table 2.1, and for the other cohort only 5% died before age one ($_1q_0$ = .05), a level not unlike that experienced by Western European populations in the 1930s when the secular decline in fertility typically came to an end. Contraceptive practice is assumed to be the same for both cohorts. If we further assume the average interbirth interval following an infant death to be 20 months, or about the average experienced by populations shown in Table 2.1, and the normal interval to be 10 months longer we can calculate the proportionate difference in the number of second and higher order births between the two cohorts. The average interbirth interval for the high-mortality cohort would be (.25) (20) + (.75) (30) or 27.5 months, and for the low-mortality cohort it would be (.05) (20) + (.95) (30) or 29.5. The proportionate difference in the number of second or higher order births occurring to the two cohorts

$$\left(\frac{\text{average interval with low mortality}}{\text{average interval with high mortality}} - 1 \right)$$

is about 7%. The difference in the total number of births would be less still, since each cohort has the same number of first births. The difference would be even smaller if we assumed the infant mortality had less than the maximum average impact of 10 months on the difference in birth intervals, which is likely to be the case in a well-nourished population. It is true, of course, that in some areas of Europe infant mortality prior to the decline was greater than the 25% assumed in our example, and in these areas the decline in infant mortality was correspondingly greater. However, high infant mortality during the last half of the nineteenth century and the early twentieth, at least, was often associated with the lack of breastfeeding or with breastfeeding of short duration (Knodel and v an de Walle, 1967). In such situations, the effect of a reduction in infant mortality would be much less than in areas where prolonged breastfeeding was universal.

Finally, we turn to the question of whether there is any internal evidence in the family history data to indicate that infant mortality affects the length of birth intervals independently of the physiological effect. One way to examine this question is to investigate the possible effect of the fate of the firstborn on the interval between the second and third births. It is evident that the death or survival of the firstborn could not affect the duration of breastfeeding of the second infant, even in areas where breastfeeding is common. However, if mortality risks among siblings were correlated with each other, there would be a higher probability of the second child dying and thus interrupting lactation if the first child died. This possible effect can be eliminated by performing calculations separately for surviving and dying second children. A relationship between the fate of the first child and the interval between the second and third births, when the fate of the second child is held constant, would be one indication of the effect of infant mortality on the birth interval independent of any effects of breastfeeding. Only one study analyzes the family history data in this manner (Knodel, 1968), but several others include sufficient data in their appendices to permit this type of tabulation. The results are presented in Table 2.2. Caution is called for in interpreting these results since the number of cases in particular categories is occasionally quite small. Nevertheless, a general pattern is evident. With only a few exceptions, the interval between the second and third birth is shorter if the first child dies in infancy than when the child survives. The impact tends to be larger when the second child survives, but it is also evident when the second child dies before age one. Furthermore, the interval between the second and third births tends to be longest if the first two infants survive and shortest if the first two die.

Of particular interest are the results from studies of families in the French village of Meulan and of the Genevan bourgeoisie, since data on these groups cover periods during which family limitation was apparently adopted by sizable portions of population and marital fertility experienced a decline. In the case of Meulan, family limitation apparently begins to be practiced among couples married between 1740 and 1789 but is considerably accelerated among couples married between 1790 and 1839 (Lachiver, 1969b). Among the Genevan bourgeoisie, family limitation and reduced fertility is apparent when the husband was born in 1650 or later

TABLE 2.2

Mean Interval (in months) between Second and Third Legitimate Confinements According to Fate of the Firstborn

| | | Second infant survives | | | | |
| | | First survives | | First dies under 1 | | |
Village or group	Year of marriage	Int.	(n)	Int.	(n)	Difference
Anhausen	1840–1890	23.4	(23)	17.6	(5)	5.8
Schönberg	1840–1890	23.9	(45)	21.1	(18)	2.8
Mömmlingen	1840–1890	29.0	(161)	25.4	(22)	3.6
Crulai	1674–1742	32.6	(129)	29.1	(41)	3.5
Tourouvre-au-Perche	1665–1765	30.4	(323)	29.8	(120)	0.6
Ile-de-France villages	1740–1799	29.3	(112)	25.2	(26)	4.1
Thézels-St. Sernin[a]	1700–1792	32.3	(79)	34.4	(8)	-2.1
Meulan	1660–1739	24.7	(232)	25.4	(69)	-0.7
	1740–1789	24.9	(208)	23.8	(51)	1.1
	1790–1839	33.3	(183)	24.1	(37)	9.2
Genevan bourgeoisie[b] Before 1650[c]		26.7	(91)	25.6	(15)	1.1
After 1650[c]		34.9	(218)	22.1	(17)	12.8
All studies	–	29.5	(1804)	26.4	(429)	3.1

Table 2.2 *(Continued)*

Village or group	Year of marriage	Second infant dies				Difference
		First survives		First dies under 1		
		Int.	(n)	Int.	(n)	
Anhausen	1840–1890	17.6	(11)	17.0	(6)	0.6
Schönberg	1840–1890	17.5	(20)	16.9	(7)	0.6
Mömmlingen	1840–1890	18.5	(27)	15.6	(13)	2.9
Crulai[a]	1674–1742	23.8	(21)	19.9	(14)	3.9
Tourouvre-au-Perche	1665–1765	19.9	(91)	18.6	(43)	1.3
Ile-de-France villages	1740–1799	24.0	(19)	20.5	(10)	3.5
Thézels-St. Sernin[a]	1700–1792	24.0	(17)	15.7	(5)	8.2
Meulan	1660–1739	21.5	(41)	19.1	(15)	2.4
	1740–1789	18.8	(37)	24.1	(14)	-5.3
	1790–1839	27.4	(21)	23.8	(6)	3.6
Genevan bourgeoisie[b]	Before 1650[c]	16.9	(20)	19.5	(1)	-2.6
	After 1650[c]	17.8	(13)	--	(0)	--
All studies	-	20.5	(338)	19.2	(134)	1.3

Sources: Anhausen, Schönberg, and Mömmlingen from Knodel (1968), Table 10; Crulai calculated from Gautier and Henry (1958), Appendix Table 8; Tourouvre calculated from Charbonneau (1970), Appendix Table 26; Ile-de-France villages calculated from Ganiage (1963), Appendix Table 3; Meulan calculated from Lachiver (1969b), Appendix Table 8; Genevan bourgeoisie calculated from Henry (1956), Appendix Table 11.

Note: In case of twins, the fate of the longest surviving twin is considered.

[a]Excluding cases where the fate of preceding birth is unknown during periods when infant deaths were incompletely registered.

[b]Excluding cases where the birth interval was estimated or where no information was available about the fate of the first two confinements.

[c]Birth years of husbands.

(Henry, 1956). In both populations, the fate of the firstborn seems to have greater impact after family limitation is firmly established than before. Such a pattern is what we would expect if the child mortality experience of a couple affects their voluntary fertility behavior.

More difficult to interpret is the finding that even during periods of assumed natural fertility the infant death of a couple's firstborn seems to shorten the time they take between their second and third births. Perhaps some voluntary control over fertility was being practiced after all. On the other hand, the small differences observed may well arise from a selection process. For example, if highly fecund or briefly breastfeeding women are more likely to experience infant deaths than less fecund women, then women experiencing infant deaths may be selected for high fecundity and therefore be characterized by slightly shorter birth intervals on the average.

CHILD MORTALITY AND THE LIMITATION OF FAMILY SIZE

The child replacement hypothesis makes sense only in contexts where couples limit their fertility after they reach some number of children they do not wish to exceed. Otherwise, childbearing would continue among all couples until one of the spouses became permanently sterile or died and would be independent of the number of children that survived or died at early ages. Any evidence of the child replacement effect operating in preindustrial European populations would therefore suggest that at least some family limitation was being practiced. Furthermore, as marital fertility declines with the spread of family limitation, the child replacement effect of child mortality on the fertility behavior of individual couples should be more apparent.

The child replacement effect should operate in such a way that the fate of the children born early in a marriage effects the couple's subsequent reproductive behavior. We will attempt to address this issue in three additional ways: by examining parity progression ratios, the age of the mother at her last birth, and the number of children ever born.

Parity Progression Ratios

If couples attempt to replace lost children, we would expect that among couples with the same number of live births (or confinements), those who experienced the death of a previous child would be more likely to continue producing children than those whose children all survived. None of the published studies analyze family history data in this way. Some approximation of the appropriate tabulation could be made based on data provided in the appendices of several of them or, in the case of several German villages, from the original data on hand. Table 2.3 presents the results, showing the proportion of women with n confinements who progress to $n + 1$ confinements according to the fate of their children. Since only infant deaths (i.e., deaths in the first year of life) were noted in the appendix tables of the French and Swiss studies used, Table 2.3 also limits consideration to experiences with infant deaths and does not take account of the deaths of children at older ages even though some would have occurred before the women proceeded to their next parities and might have influenced their behavior. In addition, for the French and Swiss studies, the fate of the last child born to each couple is not stated in the appendices, and thus the proportion progressing from parity n to parity $n + 1$ can only be related to the couples' experiences with infant deaths among their first $n - 1$ children, in order to avoid biasing the results. Since the original data for the German villages were available, this restriction was not imposed on them. For all studies, only women whose marriages remained intact when they reached age 45 (i.e., who had unimpaired opportunity to achieve completed families) were included in the tabulation. Finally, the results of any particular study need to be interpreted with caution because of the small number of cases in some categories.

The results are mixed, particularly for the cohorts for which there is no independent evidence that family limitation was being practiced (according to the original studies). Perhaps some slight tendency is apparent among these women for those who experienced infant deaths to continue childbearing than women who did not. The cohorts among which family limitation is known to be fairly widespread are of particular interest. These include couples married after 1890 in Anhausen, those married after 1740 in Meulan, and Genevan bourgeoisie couples in which the husband was born in 1650 or later. The Anhausen women do not exhibit a pattern consistent with the expectation that the child replacement effect increases as family limitation increases, but since the results are based on such small numbers of cases for the post-1890 marriage cohort, little confidence can be placed in them. In contrast, for Meulan and the Genevan bourgeoisie the relationship between the parity progression ratios and the infant mortality experience is much more pronounced among cohorts where family limitation is common. For both Meulan and the Genevan bourgeoisie, the decline in the parity progression ratios is greater at each succeeding parity for women not experiencing infant deaths.

It is worth noting in connection with Table 2.3 that a comparison of parity progression ratios by the number of infant deaths experienced could reflect the physiological effect of infant mortality on fertility as well as the child replacement effect although the impact should be slight. All else being equal, women experiencing infant deaths would experience shorter birth intervals on the average than women whose children all survive and hence would be more likely to reach each successive higher parity. For this reason, the results for Schönberg and Anhausen are particularly interesting, since prolonged breastfeeding was not common in those villages at least for the marriage cohorts between 1840 and 1890 and hence the physiological effect would not be operating. The results are rather mixed and are unfortunately based on only a small number of women. At best, the child replacement hypothesis gains only weak support from the data in these two villages. A selection process might also be operating that could give the appearance of child replacement even when couples were not attempting it. If fecundity is associated with infant mortality, then even independent of the physiological effect, women experiencing infant deaths would bear children at a faster pace than women not experiencing them simply because they were more fecund. This would then be reflected in the parity progression ratios.

Age of the Mother at Last Birth

One result of the introduction of family limitation is usually a reduction in the age at which a mother bears her last child. Therefore, if women tried to replace their lost children, women whose initial births survive childhood in populations practicing family limitation should bear their last children at younger ages than women whose first several children die at early ages. Table 2.4 presents the relevant data for the three German villages. Age of mother at the last birth is tabulated according to the number of children dying under age 10 among the first two and first three confinements. Those results should be largely independent of any influence from the physiological effect. No clear relationship between child deaths and the age of the mother at her last birth is apparent. In Mömmlingen, the relationship is in the predicted direction when the number of child deaths among the first two births is considered, but the differences are unimpressive. Even when consideration is restricted to families in which the mother was under 30 at the time of marriage, no clear relationship emerges. In addition, the relationship is either negligible or in the opposite direction among 1891–1939 marriage cohort even though there is reason to assume that they are practicing some form of family limitation. Again, we must bear in mind that the number of cases involved in this last group is very small.

TABLE 2.3

Percentage of Women in Completed Families Who Progress to Next Parity by the Number of Infant Deaths Experienced

A. According to deaths of the first n children for progression from parity n to n + 1

Village or group	Year of marriage	2nd to 3rd			3rd to 4th		
		None dies	One dies	Two die	None dies	One dies	Two or more die
Anhausen	1692–1839	89.5	97.3		88.0	92.6	(84.2)
	1840–1890	84.0	90.5		81.3	(92.9)	(90.0)
	1891–1939[a]	76.3	(66.7)		81.8		(86.7)
Schönberg	1840–1890	97.4	97.6		93.1	87.9	(76.5)
Mömmlingen	1840–1890	96.3	100.0	(100.0)	93.0	94.5	85.7
Combined German studies		93.5	97.1	94.6	91.9	92.6	84.2

B. According to deaths of the first n − 1 children for progressing from parity n to n + 1

Village or group	Year of marriage	2nd to 3rd			3rd to 4th		
		None dies	One dies	Two die	None dies	One dies	Two or more die
Crulai	1674–1742	92.6	(92.3)	--	73.8	(84.2)	
Tourouvre-au-Perche	1665–1765	84.8	94.8	--	84.0	90.4	(100.0)
Ile-de-France villages	1740–1799	90.6	100.0	--	95.7	100.0	
Trézels-St. Sernin	1700–1792	95.1	*	--	84.6	*	
Meulan	1600–1739	96.0	97.8	--	92.7	96.8	
	1740–1789	91.6	91.1	--	88.0	92.1	
	1790–1839	77.5	90.5	--	71.4	83.9	
Genevan bourgeoisie	Before 1650[b]	97.2	(83.3)	--	97.2	95.8	
	After 1650[b]	82.3	(85.7)	--	70.4	85.0	
Combined French and Swiss studies		88.6	94.7		85.3	92.6	95.0

TABLE 2.3 *(Continued)*

A. According to deaths of the first n children for progression from parity n to n + 1

Village or group	Year of marriage	4th to 5th			5th to 6th		
		None dies	One dies	Two die	None dies	One dies	Two or more die
Anhausen	1692–1839	(93.8)	85.7	86.2	91.3		84.8
	1840–1890		(88.9)	(92.9)	(100.0)		(100.0)
	1891–1939a	(90.0)	(71.4)		*	(70.0)	
Schönberg	1840–1890	(88.9)	93.1	90.9	(70.0)	85.2	80.8
Mömmlingen	1840–1890	86.1	89.3	100.0	77.7	80.4	88.2
Combined German studies	1840–1890	86.5	90.2	92.0	78.0	85.6	86.7

B. According to deaths of the first n − 1 children for progressing from parity n to n + 1

Village or group	Year of marriage	4th to 5th			5th to 6th		
		None dies	One dies	Two die	None dies	One dies	Two or more die
Crulai	1674–1742	77.4	(93.8)		66.7	(83.3)	
Tourouvre-au-Perche	1665–1765	78.2	81.2	85.7	85.7	80.8	71.7
Ile-de-France villages	1740–1799	86.2	87.2	(75.0)	90.2	83.3	(87.5)
Trézels-St. Sernin	1700–1792	(93.3)	(70.0)		(66.7)	*	
Meulan	1600–1739	87.6	82.4	(94.7)	87.5	90.0	75.0
	1740–1789	32.4	85.3	(79.6)	72.6	83.3	80.0
	1790–1839	65.1	78.8		58.8		70.0
Genevan bourgeoisie	Before 1650b	88.6	93.1		91.2	84.4	
	After 1650b	53.7	82.1		51.9	79.3	
Combined French and Swiss studies		80.7	82.7	86.0	78.4	83.1	75.2

Sources: Results for German villages were calculated for data originally collected by the author. Results for French and Swiss studies calculated from sources mentioned in Table 2.20.

Note: In case of twins, death of longest surviving twin is considered; adjacent categories are combined when either contained fewer than 10 cases; asterisk indicates results not shown for categories (or combined categories) with fewer than 10 cases; parentheses indicate results based on 10–19 cases.

a Including cases where the date of death of only one spouse known.

b Year of husband's birth.

TABLE 2.4

Age of Mother at Last Birth in Completed Families According to the Number of the First Several Children Dying before Age 10

Village	Year of marriage	Age at marriage	Among women with two or more confinements, fate of first two			Among women with three or more confinements, fate of first three		
			None dies	One dies	Two die	None dies	One dies	Two or more die
Anhausen	1692–1839	All ages	41.1	40.8	(40.5)	(41.2)	41.6	(39.7)
		Under 30	40.8	(40.7)		41.4	(39.9)	
	1840–1890	All ages	39.9	(38.6)	(40.4)	(39.3)	(39.0)	(40.8)
		Under 30	(39.4)	(37.9)	(39.9)	(38.5)		(39.9)
	1891–1939[a]	All ages	37.0	(37.2)		39.3	(38.8)	
		Under 30	36.1	(35.6)		(38.6)	(37.9)	
Schönberg	1840–1890	All ages	40.9	40.6	(40.9)	42.0	40.0	41.3
		Under 30	40.5	39.6	(39.9)	(41.8)	39.2	(40.4)
Mömmlingen	1840–1890	All ages	39.7	40.5	(40.8)	40.1	40.1	41.1
		Under 30	39.6	40.1	(40.6)	40.0	39.8	40.9
All villages[b]		All ages	39.7	40.1	40.5	40.3	40.1	41.0
		Under 30	39.4	39.6	40.0	40.2	39.9	40.6

Sources: Results for Schönberg, Mömmlingen and Anhausen marriages 1840–1890 from Knodel (1968); results for Anhausen marriages 1692–1839 and 1891–1939 were calculated from data originally collected by the author.

Note: In case of twins, the fate of the longest surviving twin is considered; adjacent categories are combined when either contained fewer than 10 cases; parentheses indicate results based on 10–19 cases.

[a]Including cases in which the death date of only one spouse is known.

[b]Including cases for Anhausen marriages 1891–1939 in which the death date of only one spouse is known.

Results from the French and Swiss studies on the age of the mother at last birth are presented in Table 2.5. Because these results had to be calculated from the appendix tables in those studies, only experience with infant deaths can be considered. In addition, since the fate of the last child is not known, the fate of the first two confinements is known only for women with at least three confinements, and the fate of the first three confinements is known only for women with at least four confinements. As with the German villages, the results are mixed, only a slightly older age at last birth being associated with women who experience the infant deaths among their first several children.

It is usually assumed that women who are older when they marry are less likely to resort to family limitation since the number of children they can bear is limited by their age (see, e.g., Wrigley, 1966). The fact that the relationship between the age at last birth and experience with infant or child mortality is in the expected direction among women married under 30 but not among women married at older ages suggests that family limitation may indeed be responsible for whatever weak relationship does exist. Further evidence of this is apparent in Meulan, where the expected relationship emerges only for the couples married from 1790 to 1839, the couples for whom independent evidence suggests that family limitation was fairly extensively practiced. It is interesting to note that the decline in the age of mothers at last birth in Meulan is greater for women who did not experience infant deaths among their first few children than among women who did. This is not so for the Genevan bourgeoisie; and indeed, for this group the relationship between the age of mother at last birth and infant mortality shows no pronounced tendency to change as family limitation becomes widespread.

Number of Children Ever Born

If couples replace children who die young, then we would expect women who experience loss of children among their first few to bear more children than women whose first few children survived. Table 2.6 indicates the mean number of legitimate confinements according to the number of child deaths under 10 among the first two and three confinements. Although the results show a mixed pattern, some tendency is apparent for women who experienced a loss among the first several children to have had more confinements by the end of the reproductive years, particularly among women married under 30. It should be noted that this relationship is not entirely independent of the physiological effect of infant mortality on fertility. Women with more infant deaths would experience shorter birth intervals on the average and hence be able to bear more

TABLE 2.5

Age of Mother at Last Birth in Completed Families According to the Number of the First Several Children Dying in Infancy

Village or group	Year of marriage	Among women with three or more confinements, fate of first two			Among women with four or more confinements, fate of first three		
		None dies	One dies	Two die	None dies	One dies	Two or three die
Crulai	1674–1742	39.7	(40.3)		40.0	(40.6)	
Tourouvre–au–Perche	1665–1765	40.4	40.2	(41.4)	40.8	40.6	40.9
Île-de-France villages	1740–1799	40.0	(39.1)		40.2	39.4	(38.9)
Thézels–St. Sernin	1700–1792	38.4	*		39.1	(40.1)	
Meulan	1660–1739	40.7	40.2		41.1	40.3	(40.1)
	1740–1789	39.3	38.8		39.4	39.6	(37.5)
	1790–1839	36.1	38.2		37.3		(38.8)
Genevan bourgeoisie	Before 1650[a]	38.9	39.5		39.2	39.3	
	1650–1699[a]				35.9	(35.6)	
	After 1699[a]	34.2[b]		35.2[b]	34.8	(34.4)	
All studies combined							
Age at marriage < 30		38.9	39.4	39.8	39.5	39.6	39.8
Age at marriage ≥ 30		41.4	40.6	40.4	42.2	41.5	(40.0)
All ages at marriage		39.3	39.6	39.9	39.8	39.9	39.8

Sources: Results calculated from sources cited in Table 2.2

Note: In case of twins, the fate of the longest surviving twin is considered; adjacent categories are combined when either contained fewer than 10 cases; asterisk indicates results not shown for categories (or combined categories) with fewer than 10 cases; parentheses indicate results based on 10–19 cases.

[a] Refers to year of birth of husband.

[b] Categories combined because of the small number of women with infant deaths among the first two confinements in each category.

TABLE 2.6

Mean Number of Legitimate Confinements in Completed Families According to the Number of the First Several Children Dying under Age 10

Village	Year of marriage	Age at marriage	Among women with two or more confinements, fate of first two			Among women with three or more confinements, fate of first three		
			None dies	One dies	Two die	None dies	One dies	Two or more die
Anhausen	1692-1839	All ages	7.0	7.8	(6.0)	(7.4)	8.5	(7.0)
		Under 30	(8.1)	8.5		9.4	(6.9)	
	1840-1890	All ages	6.0	6.9	(7.2)	(7.4)	(6.6)	(8.0)
		Under 30	(8.3)	(7.9)	(7.3)	(8.1)		(8.9)
	1891-1939[a]	All ages	4.7	(5.2)		(6.1)	(5.9)	
		Under 30	5.0	(4.9)		(6.2)	(6.1)	
Schönberg	1840-1890	All ages	6.9	7.4	(7.3)	7.3	7.2	7.7
		Under 30	7.9	8.2	(9.4)	8.2	7.9	(9.4)
Mömmlingen	1840-1890	All ages	6.6	6.6	(7.1)	6.7	6.7	7.1
		Under 30	6.8	7.3	(7.9)	7.0	7.0	8.2
All villages[b]	–	All ages	6.4	6.9	6.9	6.8	7.0	7.5
		Under 30	6.9	7.7	7.9	7.2	7.6	8.6

Sources: Previously unpublished results calculated from data originally collected by the author.

Note: In case of twins, the fate of the longest surviving twin is considered; adjacent categories are combined when either contained fewer than 10 cases; parentheses indicate results based on 10-19 cases.

[a]Including cases in which the death date of only one spouse is known.

[b]Including cases for Anhausen marriages 1891-1939 in which the death date of only one spouse is known.

children in a given span of time. Thus, the results for the 1840–1890 marriage cohorts of Anhausen and Schönberg are particularly interesting. These results are mixed and in the case of Anhausen must be interpreted with great caution because of the small number of cases involved. Curiously, in Anhausen even among the couples married after 1890, there seems to be no relationship between the number of children ever born and the loss of the first few children, even though family limitation is certainly being used to some extent by this cohort.

The results of the French and Swiss studies are presented in Table 2.7. The same constraints operate in these tabulations as were mentioned in connection with Table 2.5, since the results were calculated from the published appendix tables of these studies. Again the results are mixed but with some tendency detectable for larger mean numbers of children ever born to be associated with women who lose one or more of their first few children in infancy, particularly among women who married before they were 30 years of age. In Meulan, the association is more pronounced in the expected direction for couples who married between 1790 and 1839 than for couples who married earlier, thus suggesting it is related to the onset of family limitation. Interestingly, the reduction in the mean number of children ever born in Meulan is greater among women who experienced no infant deaths among their first few children than among women who did experience at least one infant death. Among the Genevan bourgeoisie, the association between the mean number of children born and experience with infant mortality is in the expected direction both before and after the onset of widespread family limitation. The reduction in the mean number of children born, however, is about equal for women who experience infant loss among their first few children and those who do not.

CONCLUSIONS

The limited number of studies available that provide evidence from individual data on the influence of child mortality on fertility in European populations in the past and the small number of cases involved in many of the studies make firm conclusions impossible. The difficulties are aggravated by the fact that with rare exceptions these studies did not directly analyze this relationship beyond presenting evidence of the physiological effect of infant deaths on the birth interval. Thus, much of the evidence reviewed here had to be based on a reanalysis of data presented in the appendices of several of these studies. Since these data were not presented in an ideal format for this purpose, several otherwise unnecessary constraints were imposed on resulting tabulations. Additional limitations

TABLE 2.7

Mean Number of Children Ever Born in Completed Families According to the Number of the First Several Children Dying in Infancy

Village or group	Year of marriage	Among women with three or more confinements, fate of first two			Among women with four or more confinements, fate of first three		
		None dies	One dies	Two die	None dies	One dies	Two or three die
Crulai	1674–1742	5.3		(6.8)	6.1		(7.6)
Tourouvre-au-Perche	1665–1765	6.6	6.9	(7.2)	7.0	7.3	7.5
Ile-de-France villages	1740–1799	7.2	7.5		7.4	7.6	(6.5)
Thézels–St. Semin	1700–1792	6.1	*		6.8		(6.3)
Meulan	1660–1739	7.7		(8.2)	8.4	7.9	(7.8)
	1740–1789	6.7	6.8		7.1	7.5	(6.5)
	1790–1839	5.1	6.4		5.9	6.6	
Genevan bourgeoise	Before 1650[a]	7.7	9.1		8.1	9.1	
	1650–1699[a]	4.8[b]		6.4[b]	7.1		(7.4)
	After 1699[a]				5.0		(6.0)
All studies combined							
Age at marriage < 30		6.9	7.8	7.7	7.4	7.9	7.6
Age at marriage ≥ 30		4.6	4.6		5.3	5.4	(4.9)
All ages at marriage		6.6	7.2	7.0	7.1	7.5	7.3

Sources: Results calculated from sources cited in Table 2.2.

Note: In case of twins, the fate of the longest surviving twin is considered; adjacent categories are combined when either contained fewer than 10 cases; asterisk indicates results not shown for categories (or combined categories) with fewer than 10 cases; parentheses indicate results based on 10–19 cases.

[a] Refers to year of birth of husband.

[b] Categories combined because of the small number of women with infant deaths among the first two confinements in each category.

arose from the fact that only a very few studies covered periods during which marital fertility began its secular decline. Finally, the interpretation of results was impeded by the difficulty of having to identify the influence of mortality on fertility in the presence of many other, possibly confounding, influences.

The most conclusive finding to emerge from this review concerns the impact of the physiological effect of infant mortality on the birth interval. Among preindustrial European populations, an infant death typically resulted in shortening the time taken until the next birth. Excluding the two communities studied in which prolonged breastfeeding was known to be rare, the impact of an infant death at the onset of the birth interval shortened the average time until the next birth by 2 to 13 months. Clearly much, if not all of the reduction in the length of the birth interval, can be accounted for by the fact that an infant death interrupts lactation and curtails the period of postpartum sterility typically associated with extended periods of breastfeeding. The fact that the fate of the first child was associated with the length of the interval between the second and third birth suggests that infant mortality may also exert an additional effect on birth spacing independent of the physiological effect, although the operation of some selection process could account for at least part of the observed relationship.

Evidence to support the operation of a child replacement effect in preindustrial Europe prior to the onset of at least moderately widespread voluntary family limitation was much less consistent than evidence on the physiological effect, and it is not possible to conclude that deliberate efforts to replace children dying early in life were actually taking place in most of the populations reviewed. It is interesting to note at this point that an analysis of family histories of a New England village during colonial times (not reviewed in the set of tabulations presented here) failed to show any clear evidence that couples were attempting to replace children lost by early deaths. Smith (1972) shows that among eighteenth-century women in Hingham, Massachusetts who married below age 25, there was no difference in fertility above age 30 between those women with at least one child dying before the mother's thirtieth birthday and those not experiencing any child deaths before reaching age 30 when the number of children born before age 30 was taken into account.

In the few studies included in this review that covered periods during which marital fertility was substantially reduced (presumably through the adoption of family limitation within marriage), there is some suggestion, at least in data for the French village of Meulan and to some extent for the Genevan bourgeoisie, that the child replacement effect had been set into operation. A similar finding is reported by Smith (1973) in his study of eighteenth- and nineteenth-century marriage cohorts in Hingham, Massachusetts, although his data include some anomalies. In the cases of Meulan and the Genevan bourgeoisie, declining marital fertility and the apparent strengthening of the child replacement effect appear to be more or less coincident with a reduction in child mortality. It is not clear whether either of these phenomena would have occurred in the absence of lower general child mortality. It is worth noting, however, that according to an analysis of reconstituted family histories from the English village of Colyton, a period during the latter seventeenth and early eighteenth centuries when family limitation appears to have been fairly extensively practiced was not characterized by lower child mortality than adjacent periods when family limitation appears to be absent or less extensively practiced (compare Wrigley, 1966 with Wrigley, 1968).

More significantly, the experience in Meulan suggests that once fertility begins to decline, the parity progression ratios, the age of mothers at last birth, and the number of children ever born are greater among couples not experiencing infant deaths among their first few children than among couples who lose one or more of their children in infancy. Partial confirmation of this is apparent in the experience of the Genevan bourgeoisie who show the same pattern with respect to parity progression ratios but show about roughly equal reductions in the age of mothers at the last birth or in the mean number of children ever born regardless of early infant mortality experience. Couples in the German village of Anhausen, however, do not show a similar strengthening of the child replacement effect as marital fertility declines, nor is the decline greater among couples with no child deaths among their first few children. The number of family histories that can be analyzed for Anhausen during the period of fertility decline is very small, and thus little confidence can be placed in these results.

One tentative implication of this review of evidence based on individual data for European populations in the past is that once family limitation is introduced into a population and starts to spread, couples who have unfavorable experiences with child mortality will be more reluctant than couples with favorable experience to practice birth control. Thus a reduction in child mortality should facilitate a decline of fertility. It is not clear, however, from the data reviewed if a reduction in child mortality is a necessary prerequisite for spread of family limitation. It is unfortunate that most studies utilizing family history data in the study of European demographic history have neglected to confront the question of the relationship between infant mortality and fertility beyond examining the physiological effect. The present review suggests that future research aimed directly at this problem should prove to be a fruitful area of inquiry, particularly if it encompasses the period of the transition from high to low fertility.

ACKNOWLEDGMENTS

The author wishes to express his gratitude to Nancy Williamson and Sidney Goldstein for their useful comments during the preparation of this chapter.

REFERENCES

Charbonneau, Hubert
  1970   Tourouvre-au-Perche aux XVIIᵉ Siècles. I.N.E.D. (Travaux et Documents, Cahier No. 55), Paris.
Chen, L. C., S. Ahmed, M. Gesche, and W. H. Mosely
  1974   "A prospective study of birth interval dynamics in rural Bangladesh." Population Studies 28:277–97.
Frisch, Rose E
  1974   "Demographic implications of the biological determinants of female fecundity." Research Paper No. 6. Cambridge, Mass: Harvard Center for Population Studies.
Ganiage, Jean
  1963   Trois villages de l'ille-de-France aux XVIIIᵉ siècle.
Gautier, Etienne and Louis Henry
  1958   La population de Crulai paroisse Normande. I.N.E.D. (Travaux et Documents, Cahier No. 33), Paris.
Giessler, Authur
  1885   "Ueber den Einfluss der Säuglingssterblichkeit auf die eheliche Fruchtbarkeit." Zeitschrift des K. Sächsischen Statistischen Bureaus 31:23–34.
Heer, David and Dean O. Smith
  1968   "Mortality level, desired family size, and population increase." Demography 5:104–21.
Henripin, Jacques
  1954   La population Canadienne au début du XVIIIᵉ siècle. I.N.E.D. (Travaux et Documents, Cahier No. 22), Paris.
Henry, Louis
  1956   Anciennes familles Genevoises. I.N.E.D. (Travaux et Documents, No. 26), Paris.
  1961   "Some data on natural fertility." Eugenics Quarterly 8:84–91.
Knodel, John
  1968   "Infant mortality and fertility in three Bavarian villages: An analysis of family histories from the 19th century." Population Studies 22:297–318.
  1970   "Two and a half centuries of demographic history in a Bavarian village." Population Studies 24:353–76.
Knodel, John and E. van de Walle
  1967   "Breast feeding, fertility, and infant mortality: An analysis of some early German data." Population Studies 21:109–31.

Lachiver, Marcel
   1969a   "Une étude et quelques esquisses." Annales de Démographie Historique 5:215–
          240.
   1969b   La population de Meulan du XVIIe au XIXe siècle. S.E.V.P.E.N., Paris.
Potter, R. G.
   1975   "Changes of natural fertility and contraceptive equivalents." Social Forces 54:36–
          51.
Potter, R. G., M. L. New, J. B. Wyon and J. E. Gordon
   1965   "Applications of field studies to research on the physiology of human reproduction:
          Lactation and its effects upon birth intervals in eleven Punjab villages, India". Pp.
          377–99 in Mindel C. Sheps and Jeanne C. Ridley (eds.), Public Publishes Health
          and Population Change. Pittsburgh: University of Pittsburg Press.
Robert, Patrice
   1969   "Rumont (1720–1790)." Annales de Démographie, historique 5:32–40.
Salber, E., M. Feinlieb and B. MacMahon
   1965   "The duration of postpartum amenorrhea." American Journal of Epidemiology
          82:347–58.
Smith, Daniel Scott
   1972   "The demographic history of colonial New England." The Journal of Economic
          History 32:165–83.
   1973   Population, family and society in Hingham, Massachusetts. Unpublished Ph.D.
          Thesis, University of California, Berkeley.
   1974   "A homeostatic regime: Patterns in West European family reconstitution studies."
          Paper presented for the conference on "Behavioral Models in Historical De-
          mography." University of Pennsylvania, Philadelphia, October 24–26, 1974.
Van Ginneken, Jeroen K.
   1974   "Prolonged breastfeeding as a birth spacing method." Studies in Family Planning
          5:201–06.
Wappäus, J. E.
   1861   Allgemeine Bevölkerungsstatistik, Volume II, Leipzig, Germany.
Wrigley, E. A.
   1966   "Family limitation in pre-industrial England." Economic History Review 19:82–
          109.
   1968   "Mortality in pre-industrial England: The example of Colyton, Devon over three
          centuries." Daedalus 97:546–80.

CHAPTER 3

The Role of Mortality in the European Fertility Transition: Aggregate-Level Relations

Poul C. Matthiessen
James C. McCann

In the late nineteenth and early twentieth centuries, within a time span of about two generations, the levels of fertility and mortality of the populations of Europe fell dramatically. For example, under the vital conditions prevailing in Sweden around 1870, a woman could expect to bear 4.1 children and to live 46.9 years. Around 1930, 1.9 children could be expected along with a life span of 64.1 years. Similarly, under the vital regime governing England and Wales in 1871, a woman could expect 4.7 children and 42.4 years of life while in 1931 the expectation was 1.9 children and a life span of 62.3 years (Keyfitz and Flieger, 1971, pp. 102–107). The early or predecline values of total fertility vary considerably over the nations of Europe and there is consequential variation in the postdecline values as well. On the other hand, there is relatively little movement in these values *within* European countries prior to 1870 and, in most cases, near minimum values are attained prior to the outbreak of World War II. Only France, where both fertility and mortality were in decline from pre-Napolenoic times, stands as clear exception to this generalization.

The fact that the changes in fertility and mortality are both bracketed by the same relatively brief time span has inspired persisting speculation that the shifts are causally linked. The standard conjecture is that the decline in mortality generated or contributed to the fertility transition. One line of reasoning is that the decline in fertility was, at least in part, the result of a response of couples to the improving survival chances of their children. Family size objectives could, in a context of reduced youthful mortality, be attained with fewer births. This argument appears routinely in discussions of the demographic transition and a good statement of it is provided by Carlsson (1966). Versions of the argument differ less in substance than in the significance they accord this mechanism relative to other factors bearing on the fertility decline, notably modernization and the diffusion of birth control. See, for example, Davis (1945) and Coale (1973). Another theme stresses the implications for fertility of the population pressure attending a reduction in mortality. Lower mortality implies larger cohorts surviving to adulthood and competing for scarce resources and for the means of support. They respond to this pressure by marrying later and limiting the number of children for whom they must care within marriage. For an example of this argument, see Davis (1963).

The present chapter assesses the status of these arguments and the more general statement, namely, that a decline in mortality was the initiating force in the European fertility transition, in light of the historical vital experiences of areal aggregations of the European population. Our report is based mainly on the early results of the Princeton European Fertility Project. This project was initiated about 10 years ago, and its stated objectives are "to examine in some detail the decline of fertility in Europe since the time of the French Revolution. The purpose of the project is to record the fall in the rate of childbearing in each of the more than 700 provinces of Europe in terms of a uniform set of indexes and to determine, as well as possible, the social and economic conditions under which the decline occurred (Coale, 1974)." Toward this end, several national studies have been carried out or are currently in progress. In nearly all of these studies, cross-provincial differences and changes are related to corresponding differences and changes in mortality. Detailed reports of these relations have either been published or are currently available in manuscript form for Belgium, Germany, Italy, and Portugal. Also, there is preliminary information relating to the experiences of Denmark, France, Great Britain, and Russia. We will also report on certain cross-national relations and, in so doing, we will draw on summaries of official statistics.

A major benefit of the collaborative character of the Princeton project is a general uniformity in the design and in the measurement procedures used in the national studies. In all of these studies, the fertility level of the population is assessed by the "index of overall fertility" $[I_f]$ which is the ratio of total births in an area to the number of births that would be expected if women in the province had the age-specific fertility of North

American Hutterite wives. It is computed as

$$I_f = \frac{B}{\Sigma W_i f_i}$$

in which B is registered births, W_i is the number of women in the ith age class, and f_i is the age-specific fertility of Hutterite women in the ith age class. Summation is over the reproductive ages, and the index approaches unity insofar as women in the area under study approach the extremely high fertility performance of Hutterite wives. This measure is confounded by marital composition, and, since much of our attention will be directed to differences and changes in the fertility of married women, we will refer frequently to the more specific "index of marital fertility" [I_g]. This is the ratio of the observed number of births to married women to the number that would be expected if the married women under study were subject to the age-specific fertility risks of Hutterite women. It differs in computation from I_f only in that the numerator is restricted to legitimate births and that numbers of married women are entered in calculation of the denominator. There is also general uniformity in the measurement of mortality in these studies. Except for France, all of the national studies employ the infant mortality rate as the fundamental indicator of the level of mortality. This choice is dictated in part by a desire to meet the specifications of theories that emphasize the significance of youthful mortality and in part by the fact that the materials required for its computation are generally available at the provincial level.

All of the studies in the Princeton series are aggregate-level investigations; and, as a consequence, the results may be interpreted in the same broad framework and are subject to similar qualifications in interpretation. These studies, however, are by no means similar in all respects. The statistical resources of the various nations vary in scope and detail so that analyses possible in one country are beyond reach in the others. In addition, there are differences in the statistical styles of the contributors. In this review, we will direct attention to information relating to three operational questions, each of which bears directly on standard arguments relating the fertility transition to reduced mortality and each of which is investigated in at least some of these studies. These are *(a)* Did the onset of the decline in youthful mortality systematically precede the onset of the decline in fertility in the territories of Europe and, if so, how much time typically separated the two events? *(b)* Was there a steady-state balance of fertility and mortality in pretransition Europe? In other words, is there cross-sectional evidence consistent with the view that an initial adjustment of fertility to mortality existed? *(c)* Is there evidence of an areal association in the amounts of change in fertility and mortality in the period of transition? We now take up these questions in turn.

THE SEQUENCE OF DEMOGRAPHIC TRANSITION

If a reduction in fertility is strictly a consequence of increased child survivorship, then a decline in mortality should temporally precede the decline in fertility. The amount of time required for the fertility consequences of any mortality reduction to be substantially realized should depend on the manner in which mortality influences fertility. If, for example, the fertility decline is due largely to a reduction in those births intended by couples to replace infants and children lost to mortality, the bulk of the response might well occur within as little as 2 years time. If the reduction in fertility is mainly a reaction of couples to the projected implications of improved survivorship for living or contemplated offspring, it would be reasonable to set a somewhat greater lag. This is because some time can be expected to elapse between the time that a reduction in mortality sets in and the time that its effects are appreciated among members of the population generally. While a strong basis for numerical conjecture is not at hand, it seems sensible to suggest that perhaps 5 or 10 years are required for an increased level of survivorship to become apparent in families with which couples are directly or secondarily familiar, or—as is possibly more germane—for a reduction in the virulence of any or several causes of early death to be noted and to be seen as secured. Finally, if the fertility consequences of a reduction in mortality do not fundamentally involve considerations of family replacement but stem mainly from the pressures of increased population on social institutions, a still greater lag would be anticipated. It might well require a generation for the children whose deaths were averted under declining mortality to pressure the land, the labor market, housing, and any scarce commodities for which adults compete and to so create a set of social and economic conditions that would foster a reduction in fertility.

It should be added as a cautionary note that it is possible for a mortality reduction to operate to reduce fertility without temporally preceding it. This will be true in particular when some antecedent variable or cluster of conditions diminishes both vital risks but affects fertility first. The later reduction in mortality might then act to accentuate the fertility decline. On the other hand, if reductions in mortality are presumed to be a major initiating factor in the fertility decline, there can be no escaping the inference that the decrease in deaths should stand prior in time to the decrease in births.

The early findings of the Princeton European Fertility Project do not, on face, support the notion that the transition in fertility was preceded by a reduction in youthful mortality. The results of systematic attempts to establish the temporal order of onset of the fertility and mortality declines are reported in two national studies, that of Germany (Knodel, 1974) and that of Belgium (Lesthaeghe, 1975). Knodel dates the onset of the mortality transition as the year in which the infant mortality rate declined by 10% from its maximum value. In cases in which the infant mortality rate rebounded from an early decline, the transition date is reckoned as the last year in which the rate dropped by 10% from its maximum. The date of the onset of the fertility decline is fixed by analogous procedures. It is taken as the date that the index of marital fertility $[I_g]$ fell for the last time to 90% of its maximum. Knodel reports that the mortality decline preceded the fertility decline in only 34 of the 71 administrative areas of Germany. In 36 areas, the fertility decline set in earlier, and in one case the onsets of the transitions occurred in the same year. The variability in the timing of the two transitions is underscored by the fact that an average lag of 11 years in the starting dates of the two declines is measured for those cases in which the mortality reduction occurred first and an average lag of 9 years is found for the cases in which the fertility decline occurred first. Lesthaeghe traces the paths of the infant mortality rate and the index of marital fertility in the 9 provinces of Belgium from the year 1880. In most cases, fertility is shown to be in decline from the initial year of observation, whereas infant mortality does not enter into decline until around 1895. By this time, marital fertility has declined substantially, by at least 30% in 6 of the 9 provinces. In two provinces, some parallelism in the declines is observed. However, if we follow Knodel's approach and fix the years of a 10% decline from the maximum values, we find that in both instances the reduction in fertility preceded the reduction in mortality. In only 1 of the 9 provinces of Belgium does the evidence point to the temporal priority of the onset of the mortality transition.

Commenting on the implications of the German data, Knodel (1974:185) states that "it appears that the usual description of the demographic transition which postulates a prior decline in mortality (particularly infant and child mortality) as an initiating cause of the fertility decline does not fit the facts in Germany." With respect to Belgium, Lesthaeghe (1975:11) stresses that, in general, "The drop in infant mortality occurred *after* the start of the marital fertility decline and can therefore hardly be considered as one of the factors that triggered off the trend toward greater control of fertility." Coale (1973:6), writing with knowledge of Knodel's results, assesses the implications for the European case broadly. He states that "the evidence reveals many cases in which the decline in fertility and mortality were more or less synchronous (without the postulated lag) and even a number of cases in which the decline in fertility came first.'' He alludes to France as ''the most prominent example of roughly simulta- neous declines.'' He states that ''the moderate rate of population increase [in France] in the eighteenth century scarcely accelerated during the tran- sition because the decline in the death rate during the nineteenth century was very well matched by a decline of the birth rate that occurred at the same time.'' The thrust of these results and of the observations on their significance is fundamental. If reductions in mortality did not systemat- ically precede the fertility transition, the notion that the mortality decline initiated the reduction in fertility must be rejected and the classical de- scriptive formulation of the demographic transition in Europe must be revised. Indeed, Coale is suggesting that such a revision may now be in order.

The seriousness of these implications prompts a review of the proce- dures and assumptions under which they were developed. Several prob- lems of measurement arise almost immediately. For example, what is the justification for comparing equiproportionate declines in mortality and fertility as opposed to equiproportionate increases in survivorship and declines in fertility? And why 10%? The methods used to set the date of an onset are arbitrary, perhaps necessarily so, and the very notion that any particular date has much significance in the process of fertility decline is somewhat doubtful; but, on the other hand, there is no clear alternative approach to measuring and ordering the vital transitions.

One feature of the operational procedures is more troubling—the use of the infant mortality rate to index both infant and childhood mortality. If the reduction in fertility is essentially an adjustment by couples to the replacement implications of lower mortality, then what is at stake is survi- val through childhood and not simply past the first year of life. If the effects on fertility operate through population pressure on social and eco- nomic institutions, it is survival to adulthood which is of interest. Thus, under either argument, survival to the age threshold of childhood and adulthood would seem a more reasonable index than infant mortality. Knodel argues this point fully and suggests survival to age 15 as a pre- ferred measure. He falls back on the infant mortality rate only because the data do not permit the direct calculation of a more appropriate alternative. Lesthaeghe does not discuss the indicator problem, but the theoretical arguments he reviews stress family replacement as the mechanism by which mortality influences fertility. It is fair to assume that Lesthaeghe, like Knodel, is constrained by limitations of the data. Coale's argument also stresses child survivorship.

The prevailing approach would pose few problems if there were correspondence between the timing of the decline in both infant mortality and mortality in the youthful ages generally. Since infant mortality is a large component of all mortality in the ages under 15 and since a strong positive association obtains between infant mortality and mortality in the other youthful ages, it is not unreasonable to suppose that such a correspondence existed. But the assumption does not fit basic facts in the historical record. At the national level, child mortality (i.e., mortality in the ages 1–14) generally entered decline before infant mortality, and in certain important cases this event preceded the onset of change in infant mortality by as much as a generation. Also, the early reduction in child mortality was of considerable magnitude and has a significant influence on the chances of surviving from birth to age 15. Thus, in the nations of Europe, a 10% reduction in mortality in the ages 0–14, taken in total, typically occurs earlier than a similar proportionate reduction in mortality in infancy. Finally and most significantly, the ordering of the transitions in fertility and mortality at the national level is altered substantially when information on mortality in all youthful ages rather than information on infant mortality alone is used to fix the date of the mortality transition.

The data supporting these assertions are the historical age-specific mortality statistics of 20 European nations, and these are drawn from the (unpublished) materials used to construct the regional model life Tables (Office of Population Research, no date). The 20 cases are those European nations for which mortality is observed at three different points of time prior to 1940 and for which there is at least one observation that dates to a period of high, though not necessarily pretransition level, mortality. At least one observation, that is, dates from a period in which 20% of those born died before attaining age 15. From these materials, the three life table values, $_1q_0$, $_{14}q_1$, and $_{15}q_0$, were constructed for each nation and each observation date. These values are, respectively, the probability of surviving from birth to age 1, the probability of surviving to age 15 from age 1, and the probability of surviving from birth to age 15. The measure of infant mortality, $_1q_0$, is the same as that used by Lesthaeghe and Knodel; $_{14}q_1$ and $_{15}q_0$ are, respectively, the life table analogues for child mortality and for infant and child mortality combined. In fixing the onset of changes in mortality, we determine, for each country and for each of the three parameters, the last date at which it fell to 90% of its maximum value. Knodel used linear interpolation to estimate values in the years separating his observations and we follow him in these procedures.

The first five columns of Table 3.1 show the number of dates of observation for each country, the date of the earliest observation, and the maximum observed values of each of the three mortality indexes. It is obvious from a perusal of this summary that there is considerable varia-

TABLE 3.1

Maximum Values and Dates of 10% Decline in Infant, Child, and All Youthful Mortality and Date of 10% Decline in Marital Fertility: 21 European Nations

	Cases	Earliest observation	Maximum values			Date of 10% decline			Date of 10% decline in I_g
			$_1q_0$	$_{14}q_1$	$_{15}q_0$	$_1q_0$	$_{14}q_1$	$_{15}q_0$	
France	17	1840-1842	.1901	.2043	.3567	1898	1860	1866	Pre-1830
Netherlands	9	1840-1851	.2218	.2040	.3711	1884	1873	1882	1897
Belgium	5	1841-1850	.1725	.2163	.3448	1903	1860	1871	1882
Bulgaria	3	1899-1902	.1713	.2347	.3611	1927	1903	1909	1912
England and Wales	9	1838-1854	.1771	.2120	.3409	1900	1862	1873	1892
Scotland	5	1861-1870	.1435	.2008	.3101	1904	1875	1883	1894
Sweden	9	1841-1850	.1651	.1863	.3143	1867	1869	1872	1892
Austria	4	1900-1901	.2494	.1606	.3699	1907	1907	1903	1908
Denmark	8	1895-1900	.1462	.0824	.2166	1903	1900	1902	1900
Finland	4	1881-1890	.1640	.1956	.3275	1897	1895	1897	1910
Germany	7	1871-1880	.2592	.1950	.3974	1896	1888	1890	1890
Greece	3	1920	.1137	.1785	.2719	1940	1926	1926	--
Hungary	3	1920-1921	.2152	.1601	.3408	1926	1924	1924	--
Iceland	3	1901-1910	.1207	.0943	.2036	1910	1911	1910	--
Italy	7	1876-1887	.2128	.2643	.4221	1893	1888	1890	1911
Norway	6	1856-1865	.1129	.1494	.2454	1898	1872	1880	1904
Portugal	3	1919-1922	.2349	.2112	.3965	1927	1923	1925	--
Russia	3	1874-1884	.3277	.3279	.5483	1897	1890	1896	--
Spain	5	1900	.2103	.2607	.4162	1905	1905	1905	1918
Switzerland	9	1876-1880	.2041	.1274	.3055	1884	1883	1884	1885
Ireland	--	--	--	--	--	pre-1929			1929

Sources: Knodel and Van de Walle, 1967; Office of Population Research, no date.

54

tion across countries in the depth and detail of our information. We have, in light of this, found it useful to gather our cases into three classes. The first class includes just 2 cases, France and the Netherlands. In both instances, our observations date from around 1840 and the maximum values of both infant and child mortality occur later than the earliest observation. For these 2 countries, we are in a position to determine not only which ages experienced the earlier mortality but also the difference in the dates of onset of the declines. Our second group includes those countries in which the maximum of either $_1q_0$ or $_{14}q_1$ occurs after the earliest observation. For these cases we can determine which of the two youthful age classes experienced the earlier mortality decline but can only set a bound on the gap separating the onset of the two declines. The countries in the second group are Belgium, Bulgaria, England and Wales, Scotland, and Sweden. The last and largest grouping includes the remaining 13 countries, and in these cases the maximum values of both infant and child mortality are at the first observation date. In these cases we can only fix later bounds on the dates of the onset of the mortality declines in the two age classes.

The dates of the onset of the mortality decline or of the late bound of the mortality decline are shown for infant mortality, child mortality, and for infant and child mortality combined in columns six, seven, and eight of Table 3.1. In 6 of the 7 cases in our first two categories—those cases in which we can fix the ordering of the onsets of the declines in infant–child mortality—child mortality fell before infant mortality. The length of the gap was considerable, amounting to more than 30 years in four instances (France, Belgium, England and Wales, and Scotland). The observations for Bulgaria do not bracket a 10% decline in infant mortality, and the last year of observation is 1927. Child mortality had declined by 10% as of 1903 so that there is a gap of at least 24 years in this instance. In the Netherlands the decline in child mortality occurred 11 years earlier than the decline in infant mortality. The average length of time by which the decline in child mortality preceded that of infant mortality is 30.7 years for these 6 cases. Only in Sweden is there clear evidence that the earlier decline was in infant mortality. For the remaining 13 cases, we can only fix upper bounds on the initiating points of decline, and so the patterning of dates in these cases bears only suggestively on the question of the priority of the two mortality declines. We note that in 10 of these instances an earlier bounding date is associated with child mortality and that in 2 cases the dates are the same. The number of national cases we can marshall here is small, and in many instances the historical record is brief. Still the weight of the evidence suggests that infant mortality declined earlier than child mortality among the nations of Europe.

Because of these differences in trends, a measure that comprises both infant and child mortality, such as $_{15}q_0$, tends to decline earlier than infant mortality itself. In 14 of these 20 cases, the earliest date at which a 10% decline in $_{15}q_0$ can be fixed falls before the earliest date of inferred 10% decline in $_1q_0$, and in 3 cases the declines are dated in the same year. The average lag for all 20 cases is 8.1 years. As we restrict consideration to those cases for which we have the best information, the gap widens. The average spread for the 7 cases of our first two categories, taking account of the negative contribution of Sweden, is 18.3 years. In sum, the evidence suggests that the use of the infant mortality rate to index the onset of the mortality decline in all the youthful ages systematically advances the measured date of the initiation of the mortality decline and that it frequently advances it by a considerable amount of time.

The apparent ordering of the vital transitions in the nations of Europe is affected materially by this postdating of the mortality decline. To show this, we introduce into our analysis the dates of the onset of a 10% decline in marital fertility $[I_g]$ which are estimated by Knodel and van de Walle (1967) for 16 European nations. In 15 of these cases, we have dated or bounded the mortality transition; the remaining case is Ireland. The dates of the onset of the fertility transition are displayed in the last column of Table 3.1. If we compare the dates of decline in infant mortality (column 6) and fertility for these 15 cases, we find that in 8 instances mortality fell first. Initiation of the transition in Irish fertility is set at 1929, and mortality in Ireland was near posttransition levels at this time. It is therefore reasonable to include Ireland among the cases in which the mortality decline is the earlier event, and this increases the number of such cases to 9. Still, there remain 7 instances in which the fertility transition has the earlier initiation date. The outcome is not unlike that observed by Knodel in the provinces of Germany. A comparison of the dates of the transition in marital fertility with the dates associated with the decline in all youthful mortality (column 8) yields a quite different picture. Under this comparison, there are 11 instances in which the mortality decline is the earlier occurrence, and in 9 of the cases it precedes the fertility decline by more than 10 years. Inclusion of Ireland increases the number of cases with earlier mortality declines to 12. In 2 instances the declines are dated in the same year, and there are just 2 cases in which the fertility transition preceded the mortality decline. Thus, if we take account of all youthful mortality, the weight of the evidence is in accordance with the classic description of the demographic transition: The decline in mortality set in prior to the decline in fertility.

The two exceptions to this pattern are France and Denmark, and it is of interest that in neither of these cases do the mortality statistics employed in the preceding analysis reach into the pretransitional era. As a consequence, the dates of the initiation of the decline measured with these data are only late bounds, and other evidence suggests that the transitions in mortality in these two countries actually set in much earlier. The parallel decline of fertility and mortality which Coale describes for France in the nineteenth century also holds for the late eighteenth century if Bourgeois-Pichat's (1965) reconstruction of vital rates is accepted, and so there is little statistical basis for an ordering of the transitions in that country. In Denmark, on the other hand, the supplemental evidence points to an earlier mortality decline. Vielrose (1965) lists the annual crude birth and death rates of Denmark from the early nineteenth century forward. Quinquennial averages of the death rates hover near 20 per thousand from 1840–1844 to 1875–1879 and fall irreversibly to 90% of the post-1840 maximum in 1885–1889. The crude birth rate is near 31 per 1000 from 1840–1844 to 1890–1894 and does not fall to 90 percent of its post-1840 maximum until 1900–1904, or about 15 years after the decline of mortality.

This analysis by no means settles the question of the ordering of events in the vital transition. This awaits a more systematic and detailed marshalling of the relevant evidence than we have carried out. Nonetheless, we believe that the burden of proof does not fall on those who accept the classical description of the demographic transition. We also believe that the evidence to the contrary is, in itself, too weak to discredit the notion that the transition in fertility was, in some measure, triggered by declining mortality.

THE PRETRANSITION BALANCE OF FERTILITY AND MORTALITY

The arguments we have reviewed rest on the assumption that couples curtail their fertility in response to the pressures of population implied by low mortality. If this assumption is entirely general, then, all other things being equal, the fertility of an area will be low insofar as it is subject to low mortality. In other words, a positive association between fertility and mortality should be in evidence in areal cross sections. This association should be more apparent at times when the vital rates are in equilibrium or mutually adjusted and subject to relatively little temporal variation than in periods of major readjustment such as the transitional era itself. The association should also be more visible when, as in the pretransitional era, the areal variation in mortality is sufficiently great as to imply significant differences in strategies of family building. In the current or posttransitional period, the modal expectation for a couple in virtually any area of Europe is that all of their offspring will survive childhood.

The thesis that the fertility transition in Europe was a response to a reduction in mortality does not, of course, stand or fall on the structure of relations in the pretransitional era. This thesis only requires that such a response occur in the wake of the historic mortality decline of the late nineteenth and early twentieth centuries. In other words, the "adjustment" principle need not be universal but could be conditional on the circumstances prevailing in Europe in the period of transition. There are, in addition, the standard weaknesses of a cross-sectional test. For example, to the extent that low mortality is a really associated with wealth, opportunities for migration, or other factors which would mitigate its effects, the association of mortality and fertility would be weak. Not all such factors are measurable and subject to control. For example, acceptable levels of economic and family size pressure in any region could well be defined by the long-term experience of the region, and this, in turn, could be dictated in part by the level of mortality.

On the other hand, if a positive cross-sectional association could in fact be documented, the thesis would be buttressed and no qualifications would be indicated. Such an outcome would strengthen Carlsson's (1966) assertion that couples in Europe in the pretransitional era were adjusting their fertility to external pressures, including those relating to the level of mortality.

Zero-order correlations between infant mortality and marital fertility are currently available for nine nations and regions of Europe at a point falling prior to or shortly after the onset of the demographic transition. There is, in addition, a coefficient relating life expectancy at birth and marital fertility in French departments around 1831. These are areal correlations in which provinces or other administrative entities are the units of analysis. While most of the national studies report cross-sectional correlations for several points in time, we will focus on the relationship at the earliest available date. This will place our observations within the pretransitional era or as near to it as possible. The values of these coefficients are displayed in Table 3.2. They range from $+.44$ to $-.28$, with six of the coefficients positive and four negative. Obviously, the outcome does not support the expectation of a widely prevailing positive association of the vital forces.

The hypothesis might be retrieved if it could be shown that other factors related to both fertility and mortality were, in certain of these nations and regions, acting to suppress or to reverse an underlying positive relationship. Most of the national reports engage standard ecological measures of modernization and population composition as controls in examining the

TABLE 3.2

Zero-Order Correlations of Marital Fertility and Infant Mortality and the Effects of Statistical Adjustments in Nine Nations and Regions of Europe (Earliest Historical Cross-sectional Associations)

Nation or region	Date of observation	Number of cases	Zero-order coefficient	Higher-order coefficient	Variables controlled in calculating higher-order coefficient
Germany	ca. 1880	64	.44	--	None
Portugal	1911	22	.32	.66	Illiteracy, proportion in agriculture
France[a]	ca. 1831	82	.25	--	None
Wallonia	1890	19	.22	.08	Nuptiality, secularization, literacy linguistic composition, industrialization, urbanization
England and Wales	1891	--	.08	Remains weak	Illiteracy, proportion in agriculture, proportion urban, ethnic composition
Flanders	1890	22	.08	.22	Nuptiality, secularization, literacy linguistic composition, industrialization, urbanization
Prussia	ca. 1880	34	-.04	Little effect	Urban-rural residence
Northern Italy	1881		-.26	-.09	Proportion married, ruralization, industrialization, male illiteracy, urbanization
Southern Italy	1881		-.26	-.42	Proportion married, ruralization, industrialization, male illiteracy, urbanization
Scotland	1891	--	-.28	Increases	Illiteracy, proportion in agriculture, proportion urban, ethnic composition

Sources: Knodel, 1974: Table 4.11 and p. 177; Lesthaeghe, 1975: Tables 4 and 5; Livi-Bacci, 1971: Table 43; Livi-Bacci, 1975; Tietelbaum, 1974, Van de Walle, 1974: Table 8.

[a]van de Walle uses life expectancy at birth as the indicator of mortality and the correlation obtained between this and marital fertility [I_g] is -.25. The sign is reversed in this table in order to indicate that the observed association between fertility and mortality is positive.

relationship between fertility and mortality, and this places us in a position to assess this possibility. The selection of control variables differs from study to study, but the common measures are literacy, urbanization, the extent of agricultural employment, and ethnic or religious composition. The partial correlations between infant mortality and marital fertility conditional on the maximum number of controls used in each national study are shown in the second column of Table 3.2. The control variables which were engaged are listed in the last column of the table. In some instances the results are not reported numerically, and in others the results of the adjustments cannot be summarized in a single number. In these cases, we transmit what we know of the direction and extent of any alteration of the zero-order relationship. While the introduction of these control variables does, in some instances, modify the zero-order relationship, these changes are by no means systematic. There are roughly the same numbers of strong and weak associations and of positive and negative relationships after these adjustments are taken into account as there were before. In other words, the confusing variability in the zero-order associations is not accounted for by the disturbing effects of modernization and population composition as measured in these studies.

Correlations between marital fertility and infant mortality are, as we have indicated, reported for several later dates for most of these nations and regions. While these later coefficients are, from an analytic point of view, of less relevance for the question at hand than the materials already reported, their implications should not be ignored. Table 3.3 shows all of the cross-sectional coefficients relating infant mortality and marital fertility in the nine nations and regions. Correlations of life expectancy and marital fertility in France are also presented in the table. The values shown are the highest-order measures of association that can be summarized in a single number. The leftmost value for each region is the early coefficient reported in Table 3.2.

There is a disturbing contrast between certain of these later values and the associated early coefficients. In particular, all of the four early negative coefficients are replaced by zero or by positive values at subsequent observations. The striking reversal in the two regions of Italy is particularly troublesome. The highest early positive coefficient, i.e., Portugal in 1910, is also potentially misleading. This is the partial association between marital fertility and infant mortality, net of literacy and proportion engaged in agriculture across all the districts of Portugal. The value is .66 in 1910, and the associated values for 1930 and 1960 are .33 and .85. For the years 1930 and 1960 but not 1910, Livi-Bacci (1971) reports these partial associations specific to deviations around the means of the three major regions of Portugal. Because these regions are quite different in social

TABLE 3.3

Correlations of Marital Fertility and Infant Mortality in Nine Nations and Regions of Europe (Highest Order Cross-Sectional Coefficients)

Nation or region	1830	1850	1880	1890	1900	1910	1920	1930	1940	1950	1960
Germany			.44			.30		[-.05][a]			[-.18][a]
Portugal						.66		.33			.85
Wallonia				.08	.34	.04					
England and Wales				.08		.22					
Flanders				.22	.12	-.03					
Prussia			-.04	0							
Northern Italy			-.09			.52		.58		.53	.27
Southern Italy			-.42			.33		.36		.31	.39
Scotland				-.26		.06					
France	.25[b]	.56[b]									

Sources: Knodel, 1974: Table 4.11 and p. 177; Lesthaeghe, 1975: Table 5; Livi-Bacci, 1971: Table 43 and p. 124; Livi-Bacci, 1975; Tietelbaum, 1974; Van de Walle, 1974: Table 3.

[a]Bracketed values are coefficients obtained when variables are measured as deviations from regional means.

[b]Correlations associate life expectancy at birth and marital fertility. Signs are reversed.

structure and in their cultures, this is an important control. The effect is to reduce the coefficients to the small, negative values shown in brackets in the table. It is reasonable to expect that similar consequences would attend the adjustment of the 1910 coefficient.

The net effect of these results and the associated qualifications is to weaken the notion that levels of marital fertility were adjusted to those of mortality in the pretransitional era. Strong positive associations are reported only for Germany and Portugal, and there is good reason to believe that the Portuguese relation is spurious. Furthermore, the measured association in Germany is a zero-order relation and, given the erratic response of the coefficients of other nations and regions to statistical adjustment, it cannot be accorded great weight. Modest relations are uncovered elsewhere, except in southern Italy where a fairly strong negative relation emerges after adjustment. However, the sharp temporal reversal of the Italian coefficients raises questions about the reliability of this result. It is hazardous to make universal statements on the basis of the information reported here; but when all matters are taken into account, the notion that marital fertility and infant mortality operated independently in the pretransitional era is not inconsistent with these facts.

It should be noted that this result does not compromise the general notion that a balance of vital forces existed across nations in pretransition Europe. Both the birth rates and the death rates of the nations of southern and eastern Europe were high in the nineteenth century, and both were relatively low in northern and western Europe, so that a positive crossnational association obtained. It is typically argued that postponement or foregoing of marriage was the principal mechanism through which pretransitional European fertility would adjust to changes in population pressure resulting from mortality variation, and the role of marital fertility in the adjustment process is taken to be negligible. We cannot, on the basis of present results, reject the part of this formulation that bears on marital fertility. It would be interesting, of course, to evaluate the main statement that levels of nuptiality were associated with those of mortality at the provincial level, but information relating to this question is not provided in the reports of the Princeton project.

THE ASSOCIATION OF CHANGES IN
FERTILITY AND MORTALITY

If the reductions in fertility which took place across Europe in the late nineteenth and early twentieth centuries represented adjustments to the pressures attending reduced mortality, then the magnitude of changes in the two vital forces should be positively associated. Correlations relating changes in mortality to changes in fertility are reported in three of the national studies of the Princeton project, and these provide a basis for a preliminary assessment of the notion that the transition in fertility was a response to the decline in mortality. The main results of these studies are shown in Table 3.4.

The strongest confirming evidence for the hypothesis of positively correlated changes is provided by Knodel (1974). He reports a zero-order correlation of .50 between the amount of absolute change in infant mortality between 1875–1880 and 1906–1910 and the amount of absolute change in marital fertility between 1869–1873 and 1908–1912 over the 71 administrative areas of Germany. The correlation is .45 when changes are measured in proportions. In addition, he calculates the association for 34 areas of Prussia between the date of a 10% decline in marital fertility and (a) the date of a 10% decline in infant mortality and (b) the date of a decline of .05 (i.e., 50 per 1000) in infant mortality. These measures are related to the pace of change in the two varibles. The correlation is .54 when mortality changes are measured absolutely and .38 when they are measured in proportions. Separate correlations are calculated for the urban and rural parts of the Prussian areas, and these yield coefficients of similar magnitude, though the association in urban areas is the stronger.

Livi-Bacci (1976) reports areal zero-order correlations between marital fertility and infant mortality over the provinces of northern and southern Italy in four intercensal intervals. These coefficients are uniformly small and they very in direction. He also reports the partial correlations of changes in these variables conditional on five compositional factors and, while these too are rather small in magnitude, all of them are positive in sign. Because these partial coefficients are the most refined results relating to correlated changes provided in the Italian study, they were selected for reproduction in Table 3.4.

Lesthaeghe (1975) reports the zero-order correlations between changes in infant mortality and in marital fertility in the 22 arrondissements of Flanders over the intervals 1890 to 1900 and 1900 to 1910. He does not report higher order coefficients. Changes in mortality in these two intervals are not only related to concurrent changes in fertility, but the changes in mortality between 1890 and 1900 are related to the changes in fertility between 1900 and 1910 and between 1890 and 1910. All of these associations, including the concurrent, lagged and partially lagged relationships, are positive, but all of them are weak. Somewhat stronger associations between these variables are reported for the 19 arrondissements of Wallonia in the same time intervals, but here all of the coefficients are negative in sign.

TABLE 3.4

Correlations of Changes in Infant Mortality and Changes in Marital Fertility in Six Nations and Regions of Europe in the Period of Demographic Transition (Highest Order Coefficients)

Nation or region	Interval[a]	Correlation	Control variables
Germany	M1875-1880 to 1906-1910 F1869-1873 to 1908-1912	.50(.45)[b]	None
Prussia[c]		.54(.38)[b]	None
Northern Italy	1881-1911 1911-1931 1931-1951 1951-1961	.131) .360) .397) .123)	Proportion married, ruralization, industrialization, male illiteracy, urbanization
Southern Italy	1881-1911 1911-1931 1931-1951 1951-1961	.100) .193) .032) .218)	Proportion married, ruralization, industrialization, male illiteracy, urbanization
Flanders	1890-1900 1900-1910	.168) .086)	
	M1890-1900 F1900-1910	.125)	None
	M1890-1900 F1890-1910	.100)	

TABLE 3.4 *(Continued)*

Nation or region	Interval[a]	Correlation	Control variables
Wallonia	1890–1900	−.296)	
	1900–1910	−.443)	
		)	
	M1890–1900	−.325)	None
	F1900–1910	)	
		)	
	M1890–1900	−.325)	
	F1890–1910	)	

Sources: Knodel, 1974: p. 182 and Table 4.13; Lesthaeghe, 1975: Table 4; Livi-Bacci, 1975.

[a]Intervals in which changes in infant mortality are assessed are prefixed with *M* and those in which changes in marital fertility are assessed are prefixed with *F*. If the variables are measured coterminously, there is no prefix.

[b]Changes are measured in proportions.

[c]Variables are date of 10% decline in infant mortality and date of 10% decline in marital fertility.

Taken as a whole, these results do not support strong statements. The expected positive association between changes in fertility and mortality holds rather strongly in Germany and within the region of Prussia. It also holds consistently, though weakly, in northern Italy, southern Italy, and Flanders. While an outcome contrary to expectation turns up only in the Belgian region of Wallonia, this negative result is also consistent over time and the coefficients are, on the average, of greater magnitude than those observed for Italy and Flanders. Thus, while the results balance in favor of the hypothesis of positively associated changes, the outcome is less than persuasive.

It bears noting that the measured outcome is itself subject to a number of qualifications. As explained earlier, infant mortality is a particularly weak index of youthful mortality when changes rather than levels of mortality are being assessed. All of these studies employ $_1q_0$ as the measure of mortality, and it is reasonable to conjecture that the reported coefficients are attenuated indexes of the association between marital fertility and youthful mortality. A second difficulty is posed by the fact that there are several ways in which mortality may be plausibly expected to influence fertility and that the time lags associated with these mechanisms vary. It is not unreasonable to suppose that different mechanisms will dominate causation in different territories so that the average lag will be subject to areal variation. Insofar as this is the case, any measured association of changes, whether lagged or not, will be an attenuated index of the true interdependence of the variables.

A further problem is that no statistical controls were introduced for Flanders, Wallonia, or Germany and statistical adjustment in Prussia is limited to stratification by urban and rural residence. Thus little defense can be provided against arguments that the measured associations are spurious and that they are exaggerations, attenuations, or reversals of the fundamental associations. The standard procedure of controlling for the initial levels of the change variable is employed in none of these studies. Nontrivial associations in the early levels of infant mortality and marital fertility are documented for several of these regions (see Table 3.3), and there is evidence in the reports of Knodel and Lesthaege that levels and rates of change in these variables are also associated.

These considerations should diminish any temptation to draw theoretical implications from these results. The measured coefficients are generally small to begin with, and given the possibilities for distortion, it is hard to know to what extent they reflect true relationships. Possibilities of bias are also present and there is no strong basis for assessing its direction. Thus, if the reported results favor the notion of a causal linkage between fertility and mortality, they only provide token support for it. The most that can be strongly said is that this notion is not refuted.

SUMMARY

The information reviewed does not carry us far in the assessment of the causal role of mortality in the European fertility transition. If pressures associated with the reduction in mortality played a major role in the decline of marital fertility, then certain relations in the vital forces should be in evidence at the aggregative level. In particular, the downward movement of mortality should generally precede the fertility decline, and when the variables are appropriately lagged, there should be a positive temporal association in the amounts of decline of fertility and mortality. Although the reported results of the Princeton studies support neither of these statements, slight changes in procedures produce greater consistency between results and classical theories. Whatever the association of events in the period of transition, there is little evidence of a general, positive, cross-sectional association of marital fertility and mortality in the pretransitional era. Such an association would be expected if the vital forces were initially in equilibrium; and, if this were true, a causal relation in the period of transition might be interpreted as an adjustment to a disturbance of this balance. Moreover, the information relating to this question is subject to less serious methodological qualification than that relating to the timing and association of changes in fertility and mortality. The relevant information in the national reports of the Princeton project do not point to any general, positive association of the vital forces in the years preceding the demographic transition. In the absence of such an equilibrium, any causal connection must be understood in terms of events and relations more or less specific to the period of transition, for example, the diffusion of contraception and the general process of modernization.

REFERENCES

Bourgeois-Pichat, Jean
   1965 "The general development of the population of France since. the eighteenth century." Pp. 474–506 in D. V. Glass and D. E. C. Eversley (eds.), Population in History: Essays in Historical Demography. London: Edward Arnold.
Carlsson, Gösta
   1966 "The decline of fertility: Innovation or adjustment process." Population Studies 20:149–174.

Coale, Ansley J.
  1973   "The demographic transition." International Union for the Scientific Study of
         Population. Liege Conference, Volume I, Pp. 53–72.
  1974   "The decline of fertility in Russia." Unpublished. Princeton: Office of Population
         Research.
Davis, Kingsley
  1945   "The world demographic transition." Annals of the American Academy of Political
         and Social Science 273:1–11.
  1963   "The theory of change and response in modern demographic history." Population
         Index 29:345–66.
Keyfitz, Nathan and Wilhelm Flieger
  1968   World Population: An Analysis of Vital Data. Chicago: University of Chicago
         Press.
Knodel, John E.
  1974   The Decline of Fertility in Germany, 1871–1939. Princeton: Princeton University
         Press.
Knodel, John E. and Etienne van de Walle
  1967   "Demographic transition and fertility decline: The european case." International
         Union for the Scientific Study of Population. Sydney Conference.
Lesthaeghe, R.
  1975   "Infant mortality and marital fertility decline in Belgium, 1880–1910. A short re-
         search note." Mimeograph. Brussels: Vrije Universiteit Brussel.
Livi-Bacci, Massimo
  1971   A Century of Portuguese Fertility. Princeton: Princeton University Press.
  1975   "Italy's Fertility Decline." Mimeograph.
Office of Population Research
  n.d.   Mortality Rates of National and Regional Populations. Untitled and xeroxed.
         Princeton.
Teitelbaum, Michael S.
  1974   Personal Communication to Poul C. Matthiessen, October.
van de Walle, Etienne
  1974   "Alone in Europe: The French fertility decline since 1850." Mimeograph. Prince-
         ton: Office of Population Research.
Vielrose, Egon
  1965   Elements of the Natural Movement of Population. New York: Pergamon Press.

CHAPTER 4

Estimating the Increase in Fertility Consecutive to the Death of a Young Child

Jacques Vallin
Alain Lery

A study of the relations between child mortality and family fertility may help us to answer various kinds of questions. The question of greatest immediate concern at the international level is whether a decrease in infant mortality will rapidly lead to a decrease in fertility in countries where fertility is still very high. The subject treated here concerns more specifically the low-fertility countries: Does the death of a young child lead to an increase in fertility in a population where fertility is evidently under considerable restraint? That is, does a couple losing a child tend to "fill its place"? More precisely: How frequently does a couple who would be expected to have n births in the absence of infant deaths, have $n + 1$ births when one of their children dies in infancy? The measurement of the "replacement" of death children is of interest essentially in populations with low fertility, since those not practicing birth control have no opportunity to modify voluntarily behavior that depends on the outcome of previous births. Our results, then, should help to establish the extent of replacement behavior at the end of the development scale where it would be expected to be most common.

In this paper we will attempt to measure the extent of replacement through data obtained in a 1962 French survey of family structure (Deville, 1972; Calot and Deville, 1971; Lery, 1972). This survey was carried out under the auspices of the 1962 population census. It developed a sample of 240,000 ever-married women under 70 years of age. Among them, 92,000 are classified as having achieved "completed families." These are defined as couples in which the woman first married before the age of 45 and the union was not dissolved before the woman was 45. The "number of children" of a *"famille complète"* includes only the legitimate children born before the forty-fifth birthday of the mother. In this survey, only women born between 1892 and 1916 satisfy the definition of *famille complète.* Hence, the study takes into account principally the behavior of the couples whose childbearing for the most part occurred between the two world wars. These women produced an average of 2.29 children per completed family.

For each of the women included in the sample, we know

- the year of her birth and
- her husband's social and professional status.

For every child:

- the date of birth,
- the sex,
- the birth order, and
- in the case of death, the age at death.

It is important to note that this retrospective survey has somewhat underestimated the deaths of children in early childhood. When we compare the infant mortality rate established by the survey with the one given by the vital statistics for the same period, we observe an omission amounting to nearly 30% in the category of children dead before the age of 1 year; however, this bias does not seem to be of the kind to weaken seriously the conclusions that follow.

Using the data obtained by 1962 survey, we can examine the extent of replacement behavior in two ways: (*a*) by measuring the probability that one birth is followed by another according to the death or survival of the first birth; and (*b*) by measuring the interval between one birth and the next, considering whether or not the first birth was followed by a death.

Here we immediately confront a fundamental methodological difficulty. When we compare the fertility consecutive to a birth surviving to a certain age to that consecutive to a birth dying before this age, can we attribute any difference to an increase in fertility resulting from a wish to replace the dead child? Although it is possible that the dead child died after the birth of the next one, we avoid this problem by examining the effect of child deaths that occur under 1 year of age. A more difficult question is whether the increase in fertility is really a direct product of the death. The problem is that the families in which a child dies before the age of 1 may be a nonrandom sample of all families and may, in particular, be inclined to above average fertility. One selective factor that may influence both a family's fertility and child mortality is social status. In fact, among our sample of families, infant mortality and fertility both tend to fall as social class rises, up to a certain level. We will be able to control this possible source of bias by examining the relations within a particular social class. Nevertheless, it is important to note that the families that experience infant death might still be selected from the point of view of their fertility. In this case, the measured increase in fertility would reflect this selection bias and it would be impossible to separate the effects of replacement behavior per se. Because of the possibility of such bias, our results are probably best interpreted as providing upper limits on the extent of replacement behavior in the sample.

Hence our first intention is to measure, for the different characteristics available, the probability that a dying child or a surviving child will be followed by another. Second, we study the distribution of the intervals between successive births. We conclude with a few suggestions about the desirable data needed better to study the phenomenon of replacement.

ESTIMATING EXTENT OF REPLACEMENT BY THE PARITY PROGRESSION RATIOS

Among the 92,000 completed families, we observed about 200,000 live births, of which 62% were followed by at least one other live birth. The same ratio calculated for the children still alive at the date of the survey amounts to 61%. For the children who died either before or after their first birthdays, the ratio is 74%. We can calculate an indicator of "excess fertility" consecutive to a death, which is equal to $(74 - 61)/61 = .22$, or 22% in the present case. This is only an aggregate and rough indicator of the "wish of replacement." It is, of course, necessary to apply it to groups of families as homogeneous as possible in terms of fertility. We shall obtain better precision if we proceed by birth order. In this case, the comparison is based upon the parity progression ratios, (Henry, 1972: 117, 118).

Parity Progression Ratios

We determined the proportions of women with completed families who, having borne at least n children, subsequently had another child. Table 4.1

TABLE 4.1

Distributions of Children of Rank n Deceased or Not Before Their First Birthday according to whether They Are, or Not, Followed By Another Child (Parity Progression Ratios: "Families Completed")

Birth order	Not deceased in the first year		Deceased after the first birthday (c)	Deceased during the first year (d)	General (e)	Total of the deceased (f)
	Total (a)	Not deceased at the date of the survey (b)				
Children followed by another child (1)						
1	48,132	44,899	3,233	2,827	50,959	6,060
2	28,319	26,426	1,893	1,772	30,091	3,665
3	16,367	15,369	998	1,085	17,452	2,083
4	9,643	9,080	563	691	10,334	1,254
5	5,854	5,502	352	515	6,369	867
6 or +	9,266	8,838	428	939	10,205	1,367
Total	117,581	110,114	7,467	7,829	125,410	15,296
Total number of children (2)						
1	70,267	66,163	4,104	3,336	73,603	7,440
2	49,149	46,475	2,674	2,434	51,583	5,108
3	29,033	27,630	1,403	1,610	30,643	3,013
4	16,835	16,054	781	1,018	17,853	1,799
5	9,889	9,440	449	744	10,633	1,193
6 or +	15,606	14,995	611	1,384	16,990	1,995
Total	190,779	180,757	10,022	10,526	201,305	20,548

TABLE 4.1 (Continued)

Birth order	Not deceased in the first year			Deceased during the first year (d)	General (e)	Total of the deceased (f)
	Total (a)	Not deceased at the date of the survey (b)	Deceased after the first birthday (c)			

Parity progression ratios: (1) × 1000/(2)

Birth order	(a)	(b)	(c)	(d)	(e)	(f)
1	685	679	788	847	692	815
2	576	569	708	728	583	718
3	564	556	711	674	570	691
4	573	566	721	679	579	697
5	592	588	784	692	599	727
6 or +	594	589	700	678	601	685
Total	616	699	745	744	623	744

[a] According to 1962 survey, couples in which the woman was first married before the age of 45 and where the union was not dissolved before the woman was 45.

73

presents the parity progression ratios (for the ranks $n = 1$ to $n = 6$ or more) for the following categories of children on rank n:

1. The total number of children (column e)
2. Children who died before their first birthday (column d)
3. Children still alive at their first birthday (column a)
4. Children still alive at the date of the survey (column b).
5. Children who died between the age of 1 and the date of the survey (column c).
6. The total number of children who died before the date of the survey (column f).

Category 1 (column e) gives a mean measure of the parity progression ratios for the population analyzed and therefore of the fertility of the women belonging to our sample. Category 4 (column b) represents fertility consecutive to a birth which is not followed by a death and thus gives an approximation of what fertility would be in the absence of replacement. But it probably underestimates this fertility to some extent because the families in which the child survived would tend to be somewhat smaller because child mortality is lower in smaller families. In other words, the effect of fertility on mortality is probably reflected in our figures in such a way as to bias downward this estimate when used comparatively.

It is quite the opposite for category 3 (column a), which omits the possible replacement of children who died after the age of 1, since it indicates the fertility consecutive to a birth not followed by an infant death but possibly followed by the death of a child over 1 year old. From this point of view, the truth probably lies between the two. In any case, owing to the importance of category 4 (which is included in both 3 and 1), the parity progression ratios differ very slightly from these three categories (Figure 4.1).

In the range of 68 to 69% for rank 1, they go down to 57–58% for rank 2 and to 56–57% for rank 3, and then they go up again progressively to 58–60% for rank 5 (values for the ranks 6 or more have less significance because of their heterogeneity). Fron rank 1 to rank 3, the curves indicate a decrease in fertility as the family grows larger. The rise at the following ranks reflects the growing proportion of the more fertile families among all the families analyzed in the survey.

Whatever the rank, the parity progression ratios are distinctly higher in the case of the death of the nth child than in the case where he or she is still alive at the date of the survey. But the ratios vary considerably depending upon whether the child died before or after age 1. If the child died in infancy, the parity progression ratio goes down from 85% for the first child to 73% for the second and then to 67% for the third. It then goes

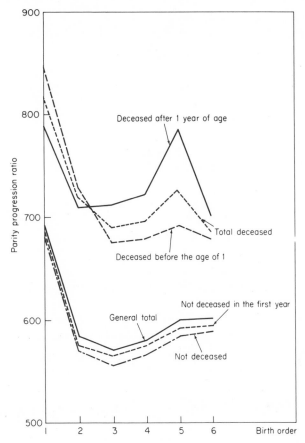

Figure 4.1.   Parity progression ratios according to the rank and the survival of the child.

up slightly at ranks 4 (68%) and 5 (69%). If we compare these figures with those obtained for the children still alive at the age of 1, the excess fertility oscillates between 17 and 26%, the maximum being reached for rank 2 (Table 4.2).

The differences are rather irregular if we compare the children of rank n deceased with the children of the same rank not deceased and still more so if we compare with this last group the children deceased after their first birthdays. In the last case, the difference works out to be 16% at rank 1, 24% at rank 2, and then 27–28% at ranks 3 and 4, jumping to 34% at rank 5. For ranks 3 to 5, these percentages probably strongly overestimate the increase in fertility we are trying to determine, because the birth of subsequent children in large families should expose earlier children to higher

TABLE 4.2

Differences between Parity Progression Ratios according to the Survival of the nth Child at Age 1

| Birth order | Parity progression ratio | | | Over-fertility | |
	nth child deceased during the first year (a)	nth child not deceased in the first year (b)	nth child not deceased at the date of the survey (c)	First measure $100[(a) - (b)]/(c)$	Second measure $100[(a) - (c)]/(c)$
1	847	685	679	24	25
2	728	576	569	26	28
3	674	564	556	20	21
4	679	573	566	18	20
5	692	592	583	17	19

mortality risks. For this reason it is much better to focus attention on the ratios given in Table 4.2. These ratios suggest that the death of a child at a young age causes an increase of 20 to 25% in fertility and that this phenomenon attains the maximum when the deceased child was the second birth.

But here we must proceed carefully for

1. In a given rank, we have not eliminated the bias introduced by selective factors that might influence both a family's fertility and infant mortality.

2. We cannot compare excess fertility of one rank with that of another. The higher the rank, the more fertile the population analyzed, hence the more limited the opportunity for excess fertility occassioned by a child death. Consequently, it is not surprising that excess fertility should diminish from rank 2 to rank 5; but this does not necessarily indicate a diminution of the wish to replace the deceased child in relation to the rise of the rank. The bigger percentage of excess fertility in rank 2 rather than in rank 1 might, on the contrary, reflect a meaningful process. The loss of a first child might lead couples to conform to the model of a family without children, whereas the loss of a second child (whose birth was the result of a wish and the possibility of having more than one child) causes an eager desire for replacement. Table 4.2 is consistent with this interpretation, but the differences are not large.

In order to avoid the first difficulty, we must make groups as homogeneous as possible from the point of view of fertility. The 1962 survey allows us at least to take account of the social and professional status of the father.

Parity Progression Ratios according to the Social and Professional Status of the Father

For each social and professional status (S), Table 4.3 compares the parity progression ratio at rank n according to the death of the child before the age of 1 or its survival at the time of the survey.[1] The differences in fertility between the different S are considerable, as reflected in the second part of the table. The parity progression ratio varies, at rank 1, from 588 for the executive staff to 775 for the agricultural laborers. Obviously, the executive staff has a greater potential to exhibit elevated fertility after a child death, and indeed this greater potential is reflected in the measure of

[1] To be exactly consistent, we should have used the same measures as in Table 4.2, by considering also the case of the children still alive at the age of 1, but the difference is so small that it seemed unnecessary to maintain the distinction.

TABLE 4.3

Probability of a Child of Rank *n* Being Followed By Another, Calculated according to Its Death Before the Age of 1 or Its Survival at the Time of the Survey, for Every Social and Professional Status

Social and professional status	Parity progression ratio										Over-fertility $[(a) = (b)] \times 100/(b)$				
	*n*th child deceased during the first year (a)					*n*th child still alive at the time of the survey (b)									
	n=1	2	3	4	5	n=1	2	3	4	5	n=1	2	3	4	5
Farmers	897	750	664	685	742	760	630	597	584	603	18	19	11	17	23
Agricultural laborers	882	801	750	806	730	775	653	638	686	642	14	23	18	17	14
Employers in commerce and industry	836	690	657	611	596	638	497	470	501	486	31	39	40	22	23
Liberal professions and managerial staff	869	679	595	452	529	679	535	529	482	508	28	27	12	-6	4
Executive staff	788	701	605	600	545	588	467	426	424	504	34	50	42	42	8
Employees	828	695	703	671	545	609	511	492	534	566	36	36	43	26	-4
Workers	829	740	677	703	711	677	582	582	588	595	22	27	16	20	20
Total	847	728	674	679	692	679	569	556	566	583	25	28	21	20	19

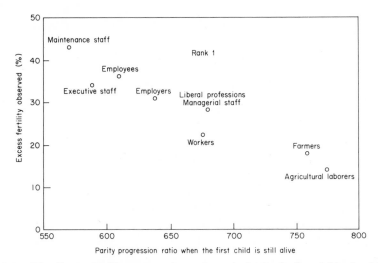

Figure 4.2. Excess fertility consecutive to the early death of a first child related to the parity progression ratio observed when the first child is still alive, according to the social and professional status of the father.

excess fertility. In general, the more fertile the wives of men in a particular class, the lower the excess fertility observed for that class. This relation is quite evident at ranks 1 (Figure 4.2), 2, 3, and 4, and if it is not true of rank 5, this is undoubtedly because of the small number of observations at our disposal at this rank (see Figure 4.3). The fact that excess fertility varies inversely with the level of fertility prevailing in a given S does not necessarily mean that the wish to replace a deceased child varies with social and professional status. The important point is that the effect of infant death on subsequent fertility does not disappear but, in fact, is maintained at about constant strength when social class is controlled.

Parity Progression Ratios according to the Sex of the Child

The sex ratio at birth is quite independent of the reproductive behavior of the couples. On the other hand, with the data at our disposal we might be able to discern the eventual effect of the sex of a dead child on excess fertility consecutive to the death. Without being able to obtain the accurate measure of replacement, we might obtain the elements for a comparison.

Table 4.4 represents the parity progression ratios according to the survival and the sex of the child belonging to rank n. Whether or not the child were to die before 1 year of age, the probability that it would be followed by another child is independent of its sex. The ratio between the two

TABLE 4.4

Differences between the Parity Progression Ratios at Rank *n* According to the Sex of the Child

Birth order	Parity progression ratio						Excess fertility (5)	
	*n*th child deceased before the age of 1			*n*th child still alive at the time of the survey				
	M	F	M/F	M	F	M/F	M	F
1	849	844	101	684	672	102	24	26
2	739	712	104	566	570	99	31	25
3	665	685	97	555	556	100	20	23
4	687	668	103	558	572	98	23	17
5	691	692	100	582	582	100	19	19
6 or +	666	694	96	586	592	99	14	17

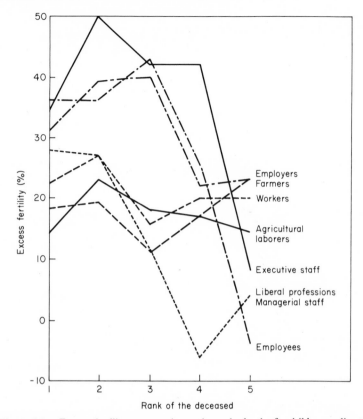

Figure 4.3. Excess fertility consecutive to the early death of a child according to its birth order and the social and professional status of the father.

probabilities oscillates between .98 and 1.02 when the child is still alive and between .96 and 1.04 when it dies at an early age. These seem to be purely random fluctuations, and if they are higher in the second case, it is because our observations are not so numerous. For the same reasons, the excess fertility indicators consecutive to the death are not significantly different whether the deceased child is a boy or a girl (Figure 4.4).

This result is not entirely devoid of interest. Although we do not know precisely what the consequences might be if couples were able to choose the sex of their children, there is no doubt that any marked preference for one or the other sex could disturb the balance of the population structure. If such a preference existed, we might expect to observe a difference in the wish to replace a lost child according to the sex of the deceased. But this is clearly not the case.

Further investigation reveals that the apparent indifference to sex of

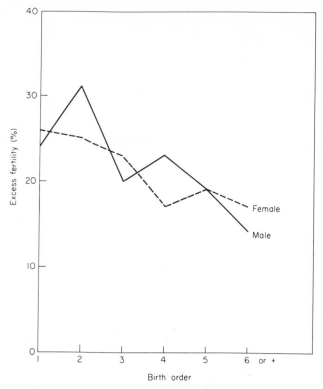

Figure 4.4. Excess fertility consecutive to the death of a child according to its rank and its sex.

children does not reflect offsetting practices among the different social groups, who exhibit essentially random behavior with respect to sex.

Parity Progression Ratios according to the Year of Birth of the Mother

The field of observation at our disposal for completed families is limited to the generations of women born in the period 1892–1916. The range is too narrow to allow an effective identification of the chronological evolution of excess fertility. But several tendencies are suggested by the data in Table 4.5. We shall discuss only ranks 1 and 2 in order to avoid categories with very small numbers of observations.

Though the parity progression ratios for ranks 1 and 2 increase noticeably in the absence of death as date of birth becomes later, the indicator of

TABLE 4.5

Probability of a Child of Rank n Being Followed by Another for Different Groups of Generations of the Mother

| Generations | Parity progression ratio | | | | | | | | | | Excess-fertility | | | | |
| | nth child deceased during the first year (a) | | | | | nth child still alive at the time of the survey (b) | | | | | 100 x [(a) - (b)]/(c) | | | | |
	n=1	2	3	4	5	n=1	2	3	4	5	n=1	2	3	4	5
1892–1899	835	699	651	647	689	658	545	540	553	586	27	28	21	17	18
1900–1904	838	698	662	684	610	659	563	573	569	595	27	24	16	20	3
1905–1909	848	750	669	690	700	669	573	561	586	585	27	31	19	18	20
1910–1914	865	749	693	686	744	709	579	553	558	572	22	29	25	23	30
1915–1916	872	812	750	714	780	734	609	550	547	558	19	33	36	31	40
1892–1916	847	728	674	679	692	679	569	556	566	583	25	28	21	20	19

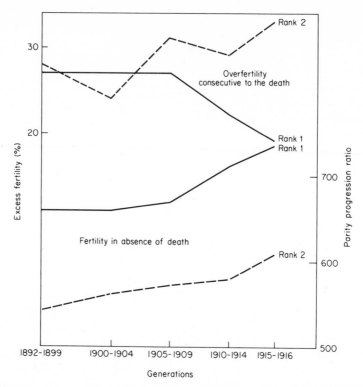

Figure 4.5. Comparison of the evolutions (according to the group of generations of mothers) of the fertility and the excess fertility consecutive to the death of a child of rank 1 or 2.

excess fertility diminishes at rank 1 and increases at rank 2.[2] For rank 1, the decline of excess fertility could be caused by the defect in the indicator that we have already underlined: its tendency to decline as fertility rises. But even though this tendency should also be operative at rank 2 (Table 4.5), the measure of excess fertility at this rank actually increases. The wish to replace a deceased child at rank 2 has increased from a group of generations to another as fertility has increased. There seems to be an increased tendency for couples who have lost their second child to refuse to accept an only child. This refusal should become more categoric in the period of increasing fertility (Figure 4.5).

[2] In France, fertility of generations was at its lowest toward the year 1895, and since then it has been increasing for the later generations coming within the field of the survey.

ESTIMATION OF EXCESS FERTILITY BY AVERAGE BIRTH
INTERVALS

We can imagine that a certain wish to replace a child deceased at an early age manifests itself by a diminution of the length of time that separates the birth of this child from that of the next. For the reasons mentioned earlier, we shall examine only children deceased before 1 year of age in comparison to children still alive at the time of the survey. After the death of an infant from illness or accident, the attitude adopted by the parents might vary according to the cause of death, the rank of the deceased child, and the total number of children they wish to have.

We have calculated the average length of closed interbirth intervals between rank n and rank $n + 1$ according to the survivorship of the child for groups of completed families characterized by the final number of children. Since the categories are homogeneous from the point of total fertility, the bias introduced by the effect of fertility on mortality is largely eliminated. Table 4.6 shows the results obtained in studying the families of two to six children. The last two columns show the absolute and relative difference between the averages indicated in columns (a) and (b).

We know that infant death occurs, on average, about 3 months after the birth in the case of the children coming within the scope of the survey. In addition to this period of 3 months (or .25 years), time is required for a couple to regain its stability and express its desire to have another child, if it has not done so before. Despite this floor beneath the birth interval, it can be seen from Table 4.6 that whatever the birth order or the final size of the family (with only one exception), the next birth arrives an average of 6 to 12 months earlier in families where a child died than in families where a child did not die. The gap is particularly long (about 1 year) in families having two, three, or four children when the deceased child happens to be the first, the first or the second, or the second or the third, respectively. When the average lapse of time is normally rather short, it cannot be reduced dramatically: This is what we observe, for example, in the case of a family of four children for the interval between the first and the second births. Even though the differences correspond rather well to our ideas regarding the objectives of the couples in planning their families, it is unwise to attribute too much significance to them because of small sample size. The relative difference is remarkably stable (between 15 and 28% of the average interval). Thus, an infant death tends to reduce the average interval between births by about 20 or 25%.

More than the difference between the averages, the differences between the distributions emphasize a certain wish of replacement, for they clearly show the diminution of the interval between the birth of the child dying in

TABLE 4.6

Average Lapse of Time between nth Birth and the Next, According to the Death of the nth Child before the Age of 1 or Its Survival at the Time of the Survey

Final number of children in the family	Rank (n)	nth child		Absolute difference (a) − (b)	Relative difference 100 X [(b) − (a)]/(b)
		Deceased under 1 (a)	Still alive (b)		
2	1	3.17	4.14	0.97	23
3	1	2.43	3.35	0.92	27
3	2	3.39	4.19	0.80	19
4	1	2.16	2.77	0.61	22
4	2	2.48	3.43	0.95	28
4	3	3.26	4.06	0.80	20
5	1	1.83	2.44	0.61	25
5	2	2.33	2.88	0.55	19
5	3	2.64	3.33	0.69	21
5	4	3.18	3.90	0.72	18
6	1	1.58	2.13	0.55	26
6	2	1.94	2.48	0.54	22
6	3	2.35	2.76	0.41	15
6	4	2.55	3.06	0.51	17
6	5	3.04	3.71	0.67	18

Note: Time values expressed in years.

TABLE 4.7

Distribution of Births of Rank 2 according to the Time Lapsed since the Preceeding Birth, Taking into Account Whether the Child of Rank 1 Is Still Alive at the Date of the Survey or Deceased Before the Age of 1[a]

	0.00-0.09	0.10-0.79	0.80-0.99	1.00-1.49	1.50-1.99	2.00-2.99	3.00-4.99	5.00-8.99	9.00-more	Total
Absolute number (1)	236	424	266	1824	1978	3184	4939	5409	746	19906
Frequency	12	22	14	96	104	168	260	285	39	1000
Absolute number (2)	25	14	25	125	131	178	184	126	17	825
Frequency	30	17	30	151	159	216	223	153	21	1000

[a] Distribution for 1000 births of rank 2, the time is expressed in terms of years and 1/100.
(1) Child of rank 1 still alive at the date of the survey.
(2) Child of rank 1 deceased before one year of age.

early childhood and the conception of the next. We have studied in detail only the distribution for families with two children (Table 4.7 and Figure 4.6). In the case of death, the distribution of rank 2 births is considerably modified: The births occur earlier than usual and the increase in natality is specially noticeable between .8 and 2 years, which was quite predictable. For example, even though nearly 20% of rank 2 births occur between the first and the second year after the first birth if the first child is still alive at the time of the survey (case 1), the proportion increases to 31% when baby dies before the age of one (case 2). The high increase in the number of births studied in the course of the first .1 years is due to the method of codification: It represents the higher mortality of twins.

Hence, the study of the distributions represented in Figure 4.6 complements the information given by the averages (Table 4.6); we have extended the study to the other categories of families and obtained very similar results.

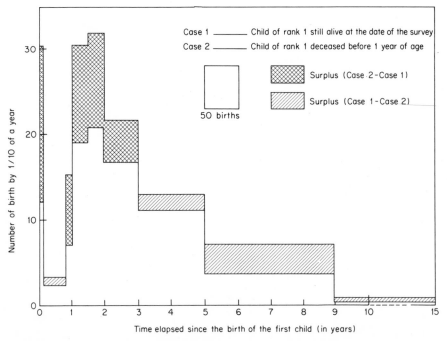

Figure 4.6. Distribution of rank 2 births according to the time lapsed since the preceeding birth (Complete families that had two children—for 1000 births of second rank).

DATA NECESSARY FOR A BETTER UNDERSTANDING OF
THE PHENOMENON

Throughout this study, we have encountered two difficulties: the effect of fertility on infant mortality; and the dependence of both fertility and mortality on other variables (birth order, S) which we would have liked to control. Both problems reflect our inability to select, for each group of families affected by infant mortality, a model group of families that did not suffer infant mortality whose fertility would match that of the first group if the latter had not been struck by any mortality.

The data used here do not permit this kind of selection. Hence, we only know that there is a phenomenon of excess fertility consecutive to the early death of a child, but we have been able neither to measure its intensity nor to make valuable comparisons between two groups (except in the case of the sex of the child and, only in part, in the case of the generation of the woman concerned).

It seems to us that it would be possible to obtain better results by constituting more homogeneous groups of families from the point of view of fertility. In particular, it would have been desirable to include information on mother's age at marriage and on the elapsed time between the birth of a given child and the birth of the preceeding one. A crosstabulation of these factors would be even more effective, but it might lead to very small numbers of observations.

We have made some preliminary tabulations of excess fertility that attempt to take these factors into account. They indicate that the woman's age at the time of her marriage does not affect the level of excess fertility, so that perhaps this factor is not a particularly important one to control. On the other hand, excess fertility varies considerably when examined in terms of the time lapsed since the preceeding birth (or marriage, if we consider the first child). The longer the interval, the higher the rate of excess fertility. This can be observed for each parity. Subsequent studies would do well to recognize this possible relationship.

We could also improve the study of excess fertility by considering the fertility that occurs after the early *death* of a child rather than after its birth. For this, we must study women of the same parity and compare the fertility without the intervention of death (or before the eventual death) with the fertility following a death, at every period lapsed since the birth of the last child. But of course this should be done for homogeneous groups of women from the point of view of their fertility. Such an analysis would seem to require a larger data set than that contained in the 1962 survey.

REFERENCES

Deville, J. C.
  1972 "Structure des familles, cuguete 1962." Les Collections de l'I.N.S.E.E., Serie D,
        No. 13/14. Paris: I.N.S.E.E.
Calot, G. and J. C. Deville
  1971 "Nytialité et fécondité selon le milieu socio-culturel." Economie et Statistique No.
        27. Paris: I.N.S.E.E.
Lery, A.
  1972 "L'evolution de la fécondité avant et aprés la derniere guerre mondiale."
        Economie et Statistique No. 37, Paris: I.N.S.E.E.
Henry, L.
  1972 "Demographie, analyse et modéle." Paris: Larousse.

Part 2

CONTEMPORARY RELATIONS IN LOW-INCOME AREAS

CHAPTER 5

The Latin American Experience

Shea Rutstein
Vilma Medica

With mortality rates intermediate between those of Asia–Africa and those of the most developed continents, Latin America is a particularly important area in which to examine the effects of mortality levels on fertility. Unfortunately, only three studies of these relations are known to the authors, and all of them have utilized areal data. Schultz (1969) and Nerlove and Schultz (1970) examined crude birth rates in regions of Puerto Rico in the period 1960–1970. DaVanzo (1971) examines Chilean regional data on child–woman ratios and age-specific fertility rates. These studies have concluded that infant mortality rates significantly influence fertility levels, and the former two attempted to identify the lag structures involved. The crude nature of the data available, however, does not permit much confidence to be attached to these conclusions. The influences of fertility on mortality cannot be satisfactorily controlled, nor can other factors plausibly considered to influence both mortality and fertility simultaneously. One of the most important of these factors in the Latin American region is differential completeness of vital registration. The implications of these studies contradict what a cursory glance at Latin American demography reveals: high and relatively constant birth rates from country to country, in the face of wide variation in child mortality rates.

The purpose of this chapter is to examine family-level relations between child mortality and fertility in Latin America. Microlevel analysis pertaining to the influence of child mortality on fertility was done using data collected in KAP-type fertility surveys in the rural and semiurban areas (areas of less than 20,000 population) in Colombia, Costa Rica, Mexico, and Peru under a program of the Centro Latinamericano de Demografia (CELADE) called PECFAL-Rural. The four surveys, utilizing standardized questionnaires and coding instructions, each interviewed approximately 3000 women of all marital statuses between the ages 15 and 49, inclusive. Information was obtained on various attitudes related to fertility, background variables, knowledge and use of contraceptive methods, marital history and, especially valuable for us, a pregnancy history, which includes information on dates of child deaths. This pregnancy history forms the basis of the data for our analysis, along with some background and other data from the survey. In all, for each country we have between 1400 and 2100 women with at least one birth on which to base our study.

LEVELS OF CHILD MORTALITY AND FERTILITY

Present levels of fertility and child mortality in the rural and semiurban areas are relatively high. Table 5.1 presents age-specific fertility rates for the 12-month period preceeding the interview, approximately midyear 1968 to midyear 1969. The total fertility rates range from a low of 6955 children per 1000 women for Costa Rica to a high of 7860 for Peru. Mexico and Colombia are about midway between the extremes.

Table 5.1 also presents infant mortality rates, calculated by the methods of Brass and Brass–Sullivan, for the four countries. These rates are lowest in Colombia and Costa Rica and highest in Peru. Using $_1q_0$ as a guide value, we see that about 15 out of 100 children did not reach their first birthdays in Peru, while in Colombia and Costa Rica the proportion is about 8 out of 100, with Mexico intermediate.

However, the rates of infant mortality do not exactly describe the incidence of the experience of child mortality on the parents. Table 5.2 presents figures on the proportion of parents who have had personal experience with a child death. Of all women who had at least one birth, at least 40% had a child die. In Peru, over half the mothers had a child die. For comparisons, we have included figures for all Taiwan taken from a similar study by Rutstein (1971). The proportion of couples there who had a child die was less than one-fifth. This remarkable difference between these Latin American areas and Taiwan is made even more notable if we exam-

TABLE 5.1

Indicators of Fertility and Infant Mortality for Rural and Semiurban
Areas of Four Latin American Countries

Indicator	Costa Rica	Colombia	Mexico	Peru
Age-specific fertility rates (per 1000 women)				
Age 15-19	105	132	115	138
Age 20-24	314	336	290	353
Age 25-29	326	331	365	395
Age 30-34	275	340	334	297
Age 35-39	207	223	247	235
Age 40-44	117	102	137	116
Age 45-49	47	16	28	38
Total fertility rate (per 1000 women)	6955	7400	7580	7860
Mean number of births				
Per woman	3.8	3.7	3.9	3.7
Per mother	5.5	5.3	5.6	4.9
Mean of declared "most convenient number of children"	5.1	4.8	6.0	5.2
Infant mortality rate (per 1000 births)				
Methods				
Brass	77.4	76.5	93.9	149.9
Brass-Sullivan	75.7	75.6	93.3	155.6
Sullivan-marriage duration	85.8	85.1	94.9	138.4
Mean of estimates	79.6	79.1	94.0	148.0

Sources: PECFAL-Rural Fertility Survey, 1969-1970. Calculation of
fertility rates for Colombia are rates of 1967-1969 from Elkins (1973),
Table 1, p. 31; and other areas are from Vila (1974), SIEF B-1.

[a]For each of the different methods, the estimates presented of the
infant mortality rates are the means of separate estimates of $_1q_0$ derived
from $_2q_0$ and $_3q_0$ using the West family of model life tables.

ine the mean number of child deaths per mother. The means for the Latin
American areas are between .76 and 1.19 deaths per mother, or from three
to five times the average for Taiwan.

The experience of child mortality is not evenly distributed. Some
women are likely to have more than one child die, especially where
mortality is high. In this respect we see from Table 5.2 that the proportion
with experience of one death is more or less constant in the Latin Ameri-

TABLE 5.2

Women with at Least One Birth according to Their Direct Personal Experience of Child Mortality, Rural and Semiurban Areas of Four Latin American Countries and all Taiwan

Child deaths per mother	Costa Rica N	Costa Rica %	Colombia N	Colombia %	Mexico N	Mexico %	Peru N	Peru %	Taiwan[a] N	Taiwan[a] %
0	334	59.2	1110	58.7	1130	54.0	890	45.3	1779	81.0
1	326	23.2	430	22.8	510	24.5	440	22.3	322	14.7
2	132	9.4	190	9.9	250	12.1	300	15.3	66	3.0
3 or more	116	8.2	170	8.6	210	9.4	330	17.1	28	1.3
Total	1408	100.0	1900	100.0	2100	100.0	1960	100.0	2195	100.0
Total child deaths	1070		1480		1720		2340		545	
Women with child deaths	574		790		970		1070		416	
Percentage of women with child deaths	40.8		41.6		46.2		54.6		19.0	
Mean number of child deaths per mother	0.76		0.78		0.82		1.19		0.25	
Per mother with child deaths	1.9		1.9		1.8		2.2		1.3	

Sources: For Latin America, PECFAL-Rural Fertility Survey, 1969-1970; for Taiwan, Rutstein (1971), Table 3.7 - KAP II.

[a]Married women 20-44 years old.

can areas at about 23%. However, the proportion with two or more deaths varies from 18 (Costa Rica) to 32% (Peru). In Taiwan, both these proportions are much lower.

Experience of child mortality is strongly related to exposure through numbers of births. Differences in the overall proportion with child mortality may be due, in part, to differences with respect to number of children born. To correct for these differences, Table 5.3 shows the figures of child mortality according to number of births (parity level). For example, from the table we see that, of women at the third parity, one half in Peru had had a child die while only slightly more than a quarter in Costa Rica had had the same experience. In the same manner, we note that at the sixth parity level over one-half of women in Peru had two or more child deaths while only one-fifth of women in Costa Rica had such experience.

TABLE 5.3

Percentage Distribution of Women by Experience with Child Mortality according to Attained Parity Level for Rural and Semiurban Areas of Four Latin American Countries and all Taiwan

Child deaths per woman	Attained parity level										
	1	2	3	4	5	6	7	8	9	10	11
Costa Rica											
0	92	82	73	64	53	47	40	38	31	23	14
1	8	17	22	28	33	33	32	31	34	30	21
2+	--	1	5	8	14	20	28	31	35	47	65
Colombia											
0	91	81	70	61	51	44	37	32	29	25	21
1	9	18	25	28	30	31	33	31	28	29	24
2+	--	1	5	11	19	25	30	37	43	46	55
Mexico											
0	88	76	65	56	47	41	33	27	21	20	16
1	12	22	28	31	33	33	30	28	29	24	24
2+	--	2	7	13	20	26	37	45	50	56	60
Peru											
0	84	65	49	38	29	20	16	9	6	4	2
1	16	29	33	32	30	28	23	19	13	10	9
2+	--	6	18	30	41	52	61	72	81	86	89
Taiwan											
0	96	90	83	76	65	56	47	--	--	--	--
1	4	9	15	20	26	31⎫		--	--	--	--
2+	--	1	2	4	9	14⎭	53	--	--	--	--

Sources: For Latin America, PECFAL-Rural Fertility Survey, 1969–1970; for Taiwan, calculated from Rutstein (1971), Tables 6.1 and 6.2.

With respect to experience with child mortality, the women in Peru are clearly in the worst position while those in Costa Rica are in the best. Colombia and Mexico, with percentages between the extremes tend much more toward the situation of Costa Rica. However, all of the Latin American areas compare unfavorably with figures for all Taiwan. Only 14% of Taiwanese women between their sixth and seventh births had two children already dead.

PATHS ANALYZED AND TYPE OF ANALYSIS

The microlevel analyses that have been undertaken involve only those paths of influence relating fertility to direct personal experience of child mortality. Indirect personal experience and societal experience were not studied because of a lack of adequate data.[1] The paths studied are both those involving family size goals and those not involving such goals.

To study the effects of child mortality on actual fertility behavior we have used as the dependent variable the parity progression ratio.[2] We believe that this dependent variable introduces the least amount of analytic bias when properly controlled for the effects of truncation and is especially useful in eliminating the effects of the reverse causal relationship from fertility to child mortality and in analyzing the effects of child mortality with respect to existing family composition. As our independent variable, we use the number of deaths of children 0 through 14 years of age that occurred before the conception that gave rise to the increase in parity. For example, if a woman had four births, her value on the independent variable would be the number of child deaths she had experienced before the conception of her fifth child. If the woman did not have another birth, then, logically, the value of the variable is the total number of child deaths she has experienced. In this way, we take into account only the situation upon which a decision to have another birth could have been based. Two biasing factors still have to be controlled for. The first of these is the truncation of length of time exposed to the risk of a subsequent birth. In other words, some women may not as yet have had another birth, although they will in the future, because the interval between these births

An attempt to use a question on the perception of changes in child mortality as a measure of indirect personal experience produced inconsistent results: Fertility and use of contraception were higher for women who perceived changes in either direction than for women who perceived no change in child mortality or could not give a reply (a substantial proportion). The variable was therefore used only as a control but no results are reported.

[2] The parity progression ratio is defined as the proportion of women having $n + 1$ or more births of those having at least n births.

was truncated by the date of interview. We have controlled for this truncation effect by including a variable representing the amount of exposure to
the risk of bearing a subsequent child, measured by the date of achieving
the parity from which the woman is progressing, in a multivariate
analysis. Also controlled are those nonintervening socioeconomic variables that are suspected of being causally related to both fertility and child
mortality.

The multivariate technique used is multiple classification analysis
(MCA), (Andrews *et al.,* 1967). This technique was selected for its ability
to handle noninterval variables and nonlinear relationships. Since MCA is
a form of dummy-variable regression, the implied model is additive rather
than interactive, but interaction terms may be included as independent
variables. The results of MCA presented in this chapter are in the form of
adjusted means of the dependent variable (fertility) for persons falling into
different categories with respect to a particular independent variable, with
the value of other independent variables statistically controlled.

Expected Results

The nonbiological paths relating direct personal experience of child
mortality to fertility depend upon the use of some form of fertility control.
We have taken the use of contraception as an indicator of the use of all
forms of fertility control within marriage since the data are unreliable on
such other forms as abstinence and induced abortion. In the areas under
study, the declared use of contraception is very low, ranging from a
maximum of 34% of women with at least one birth who have ever used a
contraceptive method (Costa Rica) to a minimum of 10% (Peru). In light of
this situation, we believe that experience of child mortality should not
have a strong effect on the parity progression ratios and that whatever
effect does exist should be greatest in Costa Rica and least in Peru.

A second expectation is that the effects of child mortality, as shown by
the parity progression ratios, will vary according to the parity level attained by the couple. Parents who have very many fewer children than
desired are likely to have another child no matter what their experience
with child mortality. In the same sense, parents who had many more
children than desired are not likely to increase their likelihood to have
another birth unless child mortality has reduced the number of their surviving children to close to their family size goals. Thus we expect that the
strength of the relationship between child mortality and actual fertility
behavior should rise to a maximum around attained parity levels near to
the mean desired family size and diminish in strength as the parity level
diverges increasingly from this mean.

Results

Table 5.4 presents the parity progression ratios (PPR) according to direct personal experience of child mortality for various levels of attained parity for each of the rural and semiurban areas included in the investigation. A comparison is made with results obtained for Taiwan using the same procedure. The parity progression ratios are adjusted for the effects of time exposure to the risk of a subsequent birth through the use of the date of the parity from which the progression is calculated (called date of previous birth for short). Additional controls used were the level of education of the woman, the quality of housing, husband's occupation, sector (rural or semiurban), and perception of changes in child mortality. The

TABLE 5.4

Adjusted[a] Parity Progression Ratios according to Experience with Child Mortality by Attained Parity Level for Rural and Semiurban Areas of Four Latin American Countries and All Taiwan

Child Mortality Experience	Attained Parity Level										
	1	2	3	4	5	6	7	8	9	10	11
Costa Rica											
0 deaths	.95	.92	.90	.88	.87	.86	.87	.81	.78	.52	*
1 death	.92	.90	.90	.92	.92	.86	.85	.81	.76	.66	*
2+ deaths	--	*	.90	.91	.90	.86	.90	.83	.84	.61	.41
Colombia											
0 deaths	.92	.90	.90	.87	.89	.83	.84	.83	.76	.66	.58
1 death	.89	.91	.90	.89	.84	.88	.83	.83	.75	.57	.54
2+ deaths	--	*	.86	.85	.84	.80	.81	.79	.75	.77	.44
Mexico											
0 deaths	.95	.94	.94	.92	.92	.91	.86	.80	.81	.80	*
1 death	.95	.92	.93	.92	.94	.90	.86	.86	.69	.63	.63
2+ deaths	--	.92	.94	.90	.93	.89	.85	.85	.76	.64	.47
Peru											
0 deaths	.92	.92	.93	.87	.80	.83	.70	.65	*	*	*
1 death	.93	.92	.92	.85	.86	.80	.75	.74	.66	*	*
2+ deaths	--	.93	.89	.87	.85	.80	.80	.75	.72	.58	.50
Taiwan											
0 deaths	.97	.91	.81	.66	.56	--	--	--	--	--	--
1 death	.98	.94	.88	.73	.70	--	--	--	--	--	--
2+ deaths	--	*	.91	.87	.66	--	--	--	--	--	--

Sources: See Table 5.3.

[a]Adjusted by MCA with the inclusion of the following control variables: date of previous birth, education, housing quality, husband's occupation, sector, fear of child mortality.

*Base less than 25 women.

socioeconomic variables were included to avoid spurious relationships since both child mortality and fertility are related to socioeconomic status.

As can be clearly seen in Table 5.4, the overall probabilities of having another birth are very high and approach those of a natural fertility population, supporting further the inference that fertility control is used very little. More important for present purposes, the parity progression ratios are scarcely affected by the number of previous child deaths. Indeed, the only increases in the PPR attributable to child mortality appear to occur in Peru, the country with apparently the least amount of fertility control, and in Costa Rica, the country with the most fertility control. A likely explanation for the Peruvian anomaly is their extended length of breastfeeding, as documented. The other two areas, Colombia and Mexico, in general show no increase and, for many parity levels show a decrease[3] when the number of child deaths increases.

In Costa Rica, it can be noted that at only 3 parity levels (4, 5, and 10) does the experience of one child death increase the parity progression ratio over the PPR for women with no such experience. At 4 other levels, one child death decreases the PPR, and at 3 levels there is no difference. Summing algebraically, the differences result in a +.14 overall increase; however, all of this overall difference is attributable to the difference at parity level 10, which has the smallest number of women. The situation is very much different if we consider differences in PPR between no experience and experience of two or more child deaths. Here we have increases at 6 parity levels, no parity levels in which the PPR decrease with increasing experience, and 2 parity levels at which there is no difference. The overall difference (the algebraic sum of the differences) is +.26. However, more than half of this overall difference comes from the final 2 parities, which have relatively small numbers of cases.

In Peru, women with one child death have higher PPR than women with no deaths at 4 parity levels, lower PPR at 3 levels, and the same PPR at 1 level. Because the elevation is in general much larger than the depression, the overall difference is +.15. It is interesting to note that in these comparisons, parity levels 9, 10, and 11 cannot be included because there are not enough women at these parity levels to permit calculation of reliable parity progression ratios for women who did not experience a child death.[4]

---

[3] This decrease may be caused in part by health problems related to the birth, causing both the death of the child and the sterility of the mother. However, it may also be caused in part by a feeling of discouragement following the child's death that eliminates the wish to have another child who also may die. This latter effect, however, presumes that contraception is a widespread option.

[4] We have taken 25 as the minimum base for the calculation of the parity progression ratios.

Comparing the PPR of women with no experience to those of women who had two or more deaths, we see that the former group has higher PPR at 4 parities and lower PPR at 2. At 1 parity level there is no difference. The overall difference is +.19.

For Mexico and Colombia, the situation is generally one of reduced PPR for women with experience of child death. For Mexico there are 2 elevated, 5 depressed, and 3 unaffected PPR for women with one as opposed to no child deaths. For women with two or more deaths, there are again only 2 parity levels with an increase, 6 with a decrease, and 1 with neither. The overall differences are −.26 and −.23, respectively, between zero and one death and zero and two or more deaths.

The situation for Colombia is similar to that for Mexico. Here there are 3 positive, 6 negative, and 2 zero differences in PPR between women with one child death and women with no deaths. For differences in the PPR between women with two or more child deaths and women with no deaths, there is an increase at only one parity level (10) and decreases at eight. The overall difference is −.25 in this case and −.15 in the former.

These parity progression ratios can be used to project the mean total additional births for women with a particular experience of child mortality. The projections calculated for each parity level are shown in Table 5.5. The calculation procedure is described in the appendix to this chapter. The present procedure is preferred to one in which the mean number of additional children actually born to the women at a particular parity is classified by their experience with previous child death. Two factors would make interpretation of the results of such a procedure problematic: The effects of truncation would be much more severe than in the case of calculating the parity progression ratios, and the results may be influenced by *subsequent* child death experience. In general, the projections show that in Costa Rica and Peru as direct personal experience with child mortality increases the mean number of additional births also increases. In Colombia and Mexico the opposite is true; increasing experience leads to a decline in the mean number of additional children. However, all but one of the increases or decreases are less than .5. Therefore, even women with the highest increases due to child mortality come nowhere near actually replacing their lost children.

PREGNANCY INTERVALS

The parity progression ratios show whether or not a woman has an additional birth; however, the rate of growth of the population also depends on the timing of births. When age at the beginning of childbearing is

TABLE 5.5

Projected Mean Number of Additional Births,[a] Total Number of Expected Births, and Increase in Projected Births

	Attained parity level									
	1	2	3	4	5	6	7	8	9	10
Costa Rica										
Additional births										
0 deaths	5.73	5.03	4.47	3.96	3.51	3.03	2.52	1.90	1.35	.72
1 death	5.73	5.23	4.81	4.35	3.72	3.04	2.54	1.99	1.46	.92
2+ deaths	--	*	4.88	4.42	3.86	3.28	2.82	2.13	1.56	.86
Increase in births										
1 death	0	.20	.34	.39	.21	.01	.02	.09	.11	.20
2+ deaths	--	*	.41	.46	.35	.25	.30	.23	.21	.14
Colombia										
Additional births										
0 deaths	5.45	4.92	4.47	3.97	3.56	3.00	2.62	2.12	1.55	1.04
1 death	5.30	4.95	4.44	3.93	3.42	3.07	2.49	2.00	1.41	.88
2+ deaths	--	*	3.91	3.54	3.17	2.77	2.46	2.04	1.58	1.11
Increase in births										
1 death	-.15	+.03	-.03	-.04	-.14	+.07	-.13	-.12	-.14	-.16
2+ deaths	--	*	-.56	-.43	-.39	-.23	-.16	-.08	+.03	+.07
Mexico										
Additional births										
0 deaths	6.69	6.05	5.36	4.71	4.12	3.48	2.82	2.28	1.84	1.28
1 death	6.39	5.72	5.22	4.61	4.01	3.27	2.63	2.06	1.40	1.03
2+ deaths	--	5.63	5.12	4.45	3.94	3.24	2.64	2.10	1.48	.94
Increase in births										
1 death	-.30	-.33	-.14	-.10	-.11	-.21	-.19	-.22	-.44	-.25
2+ deaths	--	.42	-.24	-.26	-.18	-.24	-.18	-.18	-.36	-.34

TABLE 5.5 *(Continued)*

				Attained parity level					
1	2	3	4	5	6	7	8	9	10
Peru									
Additional births									
0 deaths									
5.04	4.48	3.87	3.16	2.63	2.29	1.76	1.52	1.33	.90
1 death									
5.20	4.59	3.99	3.34	2.92	2.40	2.00	1.67	1.26	.90
2+ deaths									
--	4.66	4.01	3.51	3.03	2.57	2.21	1.76	1.35	.87
Increase in births									
1 death									
.16	.11	.12	.18	.29	.11	.24	.14	-.07	0
2+ deaths									
--	.18	.14	.35	.40	.28	.45	.24	.02	-.03
Taiwan									
Additional births									
0 deaths									
3.51	2.62	1.89	1.32	.94					
1 death									
4.08	3.13	2.32	1.65	1.28					
2+ deaths									
--	*	2.61	1.88	1.16					
Increase in births									
1 death									
.57	.51	.43	.33	.34					
2+ deaths									
--	*	.72	.56	.22					

Source: For Latin America, PECFAL–Rural Fertility Survey, 1969–1970; and for Taiwan, calculated from Rutstein (1971).

Note: Based on direct personal experience of child mortality, by parity level attained for rural and semiurban areas of four Latin American countries and all Taiwan.

[a]Calculated using parity progression ratios from Table 5.4.

*Base fewer than 25 women.

constant, the smaller the intervals between births, the smaller the interval between generations, and therefore the more rapid the annual growth of population.

An analysis using the PECFAL-Rural data of the effect of child mortality on closed pregnancy intervals was undertaken by César Fernandez (1974). In this analysis, experience of child mortality is measured by the result of the previous birth (stillbirths are excluded): still alive, died under 1 year of age, or died after 1. The dependent variable is the mean length of time between this birth and the following conception for all parity levels considered together.

The results presented in Table 5.6 show that there is a substantial shortening of the interval when a child dies before its first birthday. The decrease in average interval varies from 3.5 months (Colombia) to 6.2 months (Peru). The fact that the shortening due to a death after 1 year of age is relatively small (ranging from .1 months in Colombia to 1.5 months in Peru) implies that most of the decrease in the intervals is attributable to biological rather than motivational effects. Further support for a biological causal sequence is the observation that in Peru, the only area where a death after one year of age substantially shortens the interval, a majority of women breastfeed for longer than 1 year. It is also the only country of the four studied where a large proportion breastfeed for more than 18 months. Unfortunately, no analysis using the PECFAL-Rural data has attempted to evaluate the effect on birth timing of exclusively nonbiological influences, but study of the use of contraception provides some important hints regarding the motivational factors involved.

USE OF CONTRACEPTION

The nonbiological paths of influence depend primarily on whether or not there exists the possibility of controlling fertility. The decision to have another birth or to have that birth sooner involves deciding whether or not to use a method to control fertility. It is important, therefore, to analyze the use of fertility control methods as it may be affected by child mortality.

To study some of the effects of child mortality on fertility control, we have chosen ever use of contraceptive methods as the dependent variable and the number of child deaths experienced as the independent in the first stage of the analysis. A second stage examines when contraception began, and a third stage the continuance of use. Unfortunately, the second stage of analysis covers only Costa Rica at present. All three analyses were done using MCA. These analyses included the following control variables:

TABLE 5.6

Mean Closed Pregnancy Interval[a] by Survival of Previous Birth for Rural
and Semiurban Areas of Four Latin American Areas and Taiwan

Survival of previous birth	Costa Rica	Colombia	Mexico	Peru	Taiwan
All births	14.41	16.32	17.31	19.57	16.92
Alive at interview	14.91	16.65	17.84	20.70	17.28
Died before first birthday	10.56	13.15	13.20	14.47	11.40
Died after first birthday	14.75	16.54	17.44	19.20	17.04

Sources: Latin America, Fernandez (1974), Table 3; Taiwan, A.K. Jain
(1969), Table 1.
[a]Excluding gestation.

age of mother, total number of births, date of the last birth, marital status,
education, mass media consumption, housing quality, husband's occupation, and perception of change in child mortality. The results of these
analyses are presented in Table 5.7.

The overall percentage of mothers who have ever used a contraceptive
method varies from a high of 35% in Costa Rica to a low of 10% in Peru.
For all countries, direct experience with child mortality lowers the proportion who have ever used contraception. The largest absolute reduction,
14%, occurs in Costa Rica while the smallest, 4%, occurs in Colombia and
Peru. The largest *relative* reduction (42%) occurs in Mexico. Colombia has
the smallest relative reduction in use attributable to child mortality experience. Compared to Taiwan, the women in Latin American areas made
much less use of contraception. However, the relative reduction in use
due to child mortality is generally greater in Latin America than in
Taiwan. In interpreting these results, it is necessary to point out that we
cannot control the possibility that the chain of causation is reversed. Use
of contraception may affect child mortality through, for example, birth
interval influences on child health. It may also be an indicator of planful-
ness or concern with child welfare on the part of parents.

To see if experience of child mortality delays the first use of contraception among those who ever do use, the following procedure was used: For
each parity level reached and for each category of experience with child
mortality, the adjusted mean proportion that began to use contraception

TABLE 5.7

Results of Multiple Classification Analysis of Contraceptive Practices[a]

Child mortality experience	Percentage ever used	Mean parity level at first use	Percentage of ever users continuing use when interviewed	Percentage- using when interviewed
Costa Rica	34.6	4.97	71.7	24.8
0	38.3	5.03	73.2	26.8
1	32.2	5.70	76.7	23.3
2	29.6	5.50}		
3+	15.4	*	85.5	14.5
Colombia	19.6	--	67.1	13.2
0	20.9	--	66.6	13.9
1	17.0	--	68.2	11.6
2	20.5	--}		
3+	16.4	--}	70.5	13.2
Mexico	10.9	--	49.5	5.4
0	12.3	--	50.9	6.3
1	10.9	--	36.4	4.0
2	9.3	--}		
3+	3.8	--}	*	*
Peru	9.8	--	67.6	6.6
0	12.1	--	64.0	7.7
1	9.1	--	69.6	6.3
2	8.6	--}		
3+	7.3	--}	78.9	6.2
Taiwan	62.2	4.34	82.8	51.5
0	64.0	4.28	82.0	52.5
1	56.0	4.71	81.0	45.4
2+	61.9	4.86	88.6	54.8

Source:　Taiwan data calculated from Rutstein (1971).
*Base fewer than 25.

[a]Means adjusted for age, number of births, date of last birth, marital status, fear of child mortality, education, use of mass media, housing quality and husband's occupation according to child mortality experience for rural and semiurban areas of four Latin American countries and all Taiwan.

before the next birth, out of those who had reached the parity level without previous use of contraception, was calculated by use of MCA. From these proportions, the mean parity level at first use was calculated as the weighted average of all those who ever use.[5] The calculations reveal that in Costa Rica, experience with child mortality does increase parity at first use. The delay is approximately .7 of a child if there has been experience of one death and half a child for two deaths. A delay was also found for Taiwan.

Oddly, continued use of contraception, once that use has begun, is in general higher where there is greater experience of child mortality. Mexico, where continuance is low in general, has the only reduction in the percentage continuing contraception with an increase in experience of child mortality. Perhaps a reason for this unexpected result that continuance of use is higher among women with experience of child mortality is that fewer of these women ever use contraception and those who used it began later. Therefore these women would be more sure of what they want when they do begin and also have less chance to become disenchanted with a contraceptive technique or to encounter complications.

By multiplying the adjusted proportions who have ever used contraception and the adjusted proportions continuing such use, the adjusted proportions using contraception when interviewed were calculated and appear in the last column of Table 5.7. In the Latin American countries under study, the percentage of women using contraception at the time of interview is reduced with increasing experience of child mortality. The largest decrease comes about in Costa Rica. Usage by women with two or more child deaths is almost half that of women with no child deaths. The reduction with child mortality is more consistent in the Latin American areas than in Taiwan, where a higher proportion of women with experience of two or more child deaths used contraception at interview than women with no experience.

DISCUSSION OF FAMILY-LEVEL ANALYSIS

We have seen from Table 5.1 that the rural and semiurban areas of the two countries with the highest infant mortality rates, Mexico and Peru, have the highest fertility rates while these areas in the two countries with the lowest mortality rates, Costa Rica and Colombia, have the lowest

[5] Since the last parity level (7) included use of contraception at all higher levels, an arbitrary level of 8 was assigned. See the appendix to this chapter for the original proportions.

fertility rates. It would be incorrect, however, to attribute the high fertility of the former to their relatively high rates of child mortality without further evidence, given the two-way nature of the relationship and the various confounding factors that may intervene. It is therefore imperative to analyze the various paths of influence of child mortality to determine whether, how, and by how much fertility is affected. Of the many sources of experience with child mortality, only direct personal experience has been analyzed here.

Results have been presented to show the effects of direct personal experience of child mortality on replacement of lost children, on the timing of births, and on use of contraception. The results indicate that in only two of the four rural and semiurban areas does the probability of having an additional birth (parity progression ratios, PPR) increase with increasing experience of child mortality. In the other two areas, we have documented that there are typically decreases in the parity progression ratios. Moreover, in the two areas where there are increases in the ratios, these are small and do not occur at all parity levels. We believe that part of the reason that the PPR may decrease with increasing experience is that a woman with a child death may also have health problems that lead to both the death of the child and lowered probability of her having another birth. Since Peru has presumably the worst health conditions as implied by the infant mortality rates, the presumed depressing effect of child mortality on PPR should be greatest there and least in Colombia and Costa Rica. However, our results do not support this hypothesis. For Costa Rica and Peru, the areas with positive differences in the PPR, the increases reach local peaks around parities three to five, the numbers which more than half the women in both country areas declared to be most convenient. However, it is likely that results for Peru are strongly confounded with the physiological effects of child mortality on fertility, since breastfeeding is most common and most extended in Peru. Analysis of pregnancy intervals demonstrates that they are reduced as a result of a child death by the greatest amount in Peru.

Obviously, child mortality cannot exercise a behavioral effect on actual fertility unless the possibility of some form of fertility control exists. It is equally obvious, though, that child mortality may play a significant role in the decision on whether to use a form of fertility control or not. The decision about the use of such forms of fertility control are strongly regulated by the norms of the society. It is probable that societal experience of child mortality has played a large, if not primary, role in the formation and maintainance of such norms. Unfortunately, this process of norm formation could not be studied here.

Since fertility control within marriage is necessary for a behavioral response in actual fertility to direct personal experience of child mortality, it could be a precursor to such a response. Evidence of differences in control according to child mortality experience may indicate the beginning of such behavioral responses, even though changes in actual fertility may not yet have occurred. It is in this sense that the relationships between child mortality and the use of contraception are examined.

In general, it was found that direct experience with child mortality decreases the proportion of families who have decided to use a contraceptive method and, at least in Costa Rica, postpones the beginning of use for those that do decide to use. There is evidence, however, that once women with child mortality do begin use of contraception they are more likely to continue using it. The overall result is that among women at a certain age and parity at time of interview, those with experience of child mortality are slightly less likely to be using a contraceptive method.

In summary, we conclude that where it exists, that is in Peru and Costa Rica, the increase in actual fertility as a response to direct experience of child mortality is small, much less than that necessary for the replacement of lost children. The small response is to be expected, given the low overall levels of contraceptive use in these areas. There is some indication from the results obtained on contraception that as the knowledge and materials of contraception become widespread, direct experience of child mortality may in the near future begin to affect fertility levels in those countries, Mexico and Colombia, that have as not yet shown such effects. But it is likely that under present circumstances, further decreases in child mortality in these areas would be little offset by decreases in fertility through the mechanism of direct personal experience. Therefore, unless reductions in indirect personal experience and societal experience bring sufficient concomitant decreases in fertility, such a mortality decrease would create substantial increases in the rate of population growth. Further investigation into the existence and time lags of these other paths of influence is strongly needed.

APPENDIX: PROCEDURES FOR CALCULATING PROJECTED NUMBER OF ADDITIONAL BIRTHS

Expected Additional Births

The calculation of the number of expected additional births from parity progression ratios is a procedure analogous to the calculation of life expectancy in a life table. The formula

$$w_x = \prod_{i=1}^{x-1} p_i$$

gives the number of women reaching a parity level x, w_x (corresponding to l_x), as the product of the parity progression ratio at each level, p_i, up to level x (corresponding to $1 - q_x$).

Summing from below, the expression

$$S_x = \sum_{i=x+1}^{n} w_i \qquad (n = \text{last level considered})$$

then gives the number of additional women-levels attained, S_x, (corresponding to T_x) by women reaching level x. Dividing each S_x by the corresponding w_x gives the expected number of additional births for women attaining parity level x. These computations were performed separately for women with a particular experience with child mortality.

In the few cases at the highest parity levels, where the PPR were not available separately by number of deaths because of a small number of cases, the overall PPR for the level was used instead.

Time of First Use of Contraception

A somewhat similar procedure was used to calculate the mean parity level at first use of contraception. If p_x is the proportion of women beginning use of contraception between parities x and $x + 1$, then

$$NU_x = \prod_{j=1}^{x} (1 - p_j)$$

is the proportion of never users at parity level x. The mean parity at first use for ever users, *MPFU,* is given by

$$MPFU = \frac{\sum_{x=1}^{n} (1 - NU_x) \cdot x}{\sum_{x'=1}^{n} (1 - NU_x)}$$

where n is the last level used in the calculation. Since p_{7+} pertains to all women above the seventh parity level, we have arbitrarily chosen a value of 8 to use in the calculation.

REFERENCES

Andrews, Frank, James Morgan and John Sonquist
  1967   Multiple Classification Analysis. Michigan: Institute for Social Research, University of Michigan.
DaVanzo, Julie
  1971   The Determinants of Family Formation in Chile—1960. Santa Monica, California: Rand, R-830-AID.
Elkins, Henry
  1973   "Cambio de fecundidad en Colombia." In La fecundidad en Colombia, ASCOFAME. Fernandez, César
Fernández, César
  1974   Factores que influyen en los intervalos intergenésicos de mujeres que viven en zonas rurales y semiurbanas de América Latina. Santiago: CELADE, SIEF B-1.
Jain, A. K.
  1969   "Pregnancy outcome and the time required for next conception." Population Studies 23:423.
Nerlove, Marc and T. Paul Schultz
  1970   Love and life between the censuses: A model of family planning decision making in Puerto Rico. 1950–1960. Santa Monica, California: RAND, RM-6322-AID.
Rutstein, Shea Oscar
  1971   The influence of child mortality on fertility in Taiwan. Unpublished doctoral dissertation, University of Michigan.
Schultz, T. Paul
  1969   "An economic model of family planning and fertility." Journal of Political Economy 77:153–80.
Sullivan, Jeremiah
  1972   "Models for the estimation of the probability of dying between birth and exact ages of early childhood." Population Studies 26:79–98.
Vila, Claudio
  1974   CELADE, SIEF B-1 (unpublished).

CHAPTER 6

Experience in Pakistan and Bangladesh

A. K. M. Alauddin Chowdhury
Atiqur Rahman Khan
Lincoln C. Chen

The relationship between mortality and fertility is one of the most significant areas of policy-oriented population research. Indeed, knowledge regarding one aspect of this complex relationship has already proven to be useful in shaping population policy. In the past two decades, the adoption and implementation of many national family planning programs, despite potential opposition, have been based, at least in part, on research documenting the adverse consequences of excessively high fertility on child health and mortality (Wray, 1971; Nortman, 1974). Such information has also provided a key policy rationale for the participation of health scientists, administrators, and health ministries in population control programs.

Research regarding the reverse relationship, the consequences of mortality for fertility, however, is much less conclusive. Some have argued that child mortality experience is an important determinant of fertility and therefore the reduction of child mortality may be a precondition for successful population control efforts. It follows that population resources directed toward achieving demographic goals may be invested with high cost effectiveness in mortality control programs (WHO).

Substantive support for such conclusions, it is argued, comes from research validating the "child survival hypothesis." This term has been used to denote various proposals regarding the effect of mortality on reproductive attitudes and behavior. Poor child survivorship, it is proposed, inflates desired family size, causes couples to overcompensate by exceeding their reproductive goals, and acts as a barrier to contraceptive practice (Taylor and Hall, 1967; Omran, 1971). These effects of mortality on reproductive behavior conceivably may operate at either the community (macro) or individual (micro) levels (Heer and Wu, 1975). At the community level, child mortality experience may shape the reproductive norms and behavior of a community overall, while among individual couples, previous child deaths may affect fertility differentials between individual couples. These effects obviously need not be mutually exclusive; if present, they would be expected to reinforce each other.

Previous investigations on the child survival hypothesis have been conducted at both macrolevel and microlevel. Using cross-sectional data, several investigators have reported that lower regional death rates are correlated with lower levels of fertility or that the decline of the death rate when lagged several years has substantial negative effects on the birth rate (Schultz, 1966; Nerlove and Schultz, 1970). One difficulty with these macrostudies, however, is an inability to isolate the effect of mortality on fertility or other confounding variables. Correlations of these two variables between regions or communities could be attributed to the well documented reverse effects of high fertility on mortality. Most researchers have therefore focused on the microlevel, studying the differential fertility of individual couples according to child mortality experience. Commonly employing retrospective pregnancy histories, several researchers in Egypt, Turkey, India, and Taiwan have found higher fertility among women with previous child deaths in comparison with women with no child death experiences (Hassan, 1966; Adlakha, 1970; Wyon and Gordon, 1972; Harrington, 1971). These investigators concluded that the observed differentials in fertility were attributable to a child-replacement motivational response on the part of women with child death experiences.

But the reproductive consequences of child loss need not be simply attitudinal and behavioral. Death of infants may also abbreviate postpartum lactational amenorrhea, a period of temporary sterility, thereby exposing a woman to earlier risk of conception than she would have experienced if the child had survived. Breastfeeding is nearly universal in the rural areas of low-income countries, and cessation of breastfeeding has been shown to have profound effects on fertility (Jalliffe, 1968; Tietze, 1961; Potter et al., 1965). Many previous researchers have neglected to control for this biological mechanism, and those who have recognized this difficulty have rarely been able to adequately isolate behavioral from biological mechanisms.

This chapter presents an empirical analysis of the effects, both behavioral and biological, of child mortality experience on subsequent fertility in two predominately Islamic South Asian cultures with moderately high levels of child mortality. Data for the investigation come from two sources: retrospective pregnancy histories of a national probability sample of currently married women interviewed in the Pakistan National Impact Survey (Government of Pakistan, 1974) and longitudinal vital registration data of rural women followed from 1966 to 1970 by the Cholera Research Laboratory (CRL) in a rural population laboratory in Bangladesh (Mosley et al., 1970). The analysis attempts to illustrate how inadequate methodological treatment of data may lead to conflicting results, to distinguish behavioral effects from biological influences, to quantify the relative magnitude of these two mechanisms, and to discuss the implication of these research findings for future research.

DATA SOURCES AND METHODS

Table 6.1 presents some selected characteristics of the two sets of data employed in this study. The Pakistan data come from the National Impact Survey conducted in 1968–1969. The survey was an extended KAP type of survey containing detailed information regarding retrospective pregnancy histories, demographic and socioeconomic characteristics, and family planning knowledge, attitude, and practice of female respondents. The sampling frame of the survey consisted of all households in Pakistan (formerly the West Wing of Pakistan) excluding tribal areas. A national probability sample was obtained by a two-stage procedure, stratifying for urban and rural residence. Altogether about 2500 households were selected. This chapter examines the reproductive pattern of 2910 currently married women under the ages of 55 years interviewed in the selected households. To minimize errors introduced by recall lapse of

TABLE 6.1

Selected Characteristics of the Pakistan and Bangladesh Studies

Study characteristics	Pakistan	Bangladesh
Methodology	Retrospective	Prospective
Population	National sample	Regional sample
Residence	Urban-Rural	Rural
Sample size	2910	5236
Time covered	1960-1968	1966-1970

distant events, only pregnancy histories from 1960 to 1968 are considered in this analysis. More extensive discussions of the methodology and validity of the impact survey data have been reported elsewhere (Government of Pakistan, 1974).

The Bangladesh data come from the vital registration system maintained by the Cholera Research Laboratory (CRL) in a rural population of about 120,000 persons residing in Matlab thana, Comilla District. A census of this population was completed early in 1966; and beginning on May 1, 1966, the registration of all births, deaths, and migrations was instituted by trained CRL field staff. Detailed information regarding the CRL data collection procedures has been reported earlier (Mosley *et al.*, 1970; Stoeckel *et al.*, 1972; Chen *et al.*, 1974). The data employed in this investigation come from longitudinal observation of 5263 women who delivered a live birth between May 1, 1966 and April 30, 1967. Reports of subsequent births and child deaths occurring to these women and their children during a four-year period of observation, May 1, 1966 to April 30, 1970, were matched by computer. This represented an average observation period of 42 months per woman. Because of coding, punching, and matching errors, however, 27 cases were excluded from this study. The analysis therefore is confined to 5236 women about whom there is reasonably complete information.

Despite the differing nature of the data from Pakistan (retrospective) and Bangladesh (prospective), an attempt is made here to treat these data in a similar methodological fashion. The data are examined with respect to the illumination they can provide on the dynamics of interbirth intervals (Henry, 1961; Perrin and Sheps, 1964; Potter, 1963). A birth interval is simply the time between successive births. After a pregnancy termination, a woman typically experiences a period of temporary sterility, characterized by postpartum amenorrhea. With the onset of postpartum menses and ovulation, the woman again becomes at risk to pregnancy. This period is terminated by a conception, which marks the beginning of gestation. At the completion of the pregnancy, one birth interval is completed and another has begun. The length of an average birth interval is important because it is a direct measure of fertility. Birth interval lengths are inversely related to fertility; long intervals are associated with low fertility and vice versa.

Because of probable underreporting and underregistration of fetal wastages, only intervals between live births are considered in this study. Two types of birth interval data are presented. The first are mean intervals from one live birth to the next. These are computed by simply averaging all intervals where a live birth has been followed by another during the period of observation. Mean intervals are biased toward brevity since intervals where a live birth is not followed by another during the observation period (longer intervals) are excluded. This bias is minimized by employing life tables to compute median birth intervals. The life table technique, as employed by Potter, considers all intervals regardless of whether they terminate or not during the period of observation (Potter *et al.*, 1965). The Appendix at the end of this chapter contains an illustrative computation of a life table of live-birth to live-birth intervals during 1960–1968 for parity 1 Pakistani women who had no previous child deaths.

For the Bangladesh prospective data, the beginning of all intervals was marked by the live birth event in 1966–1967 (parity i birth). Women then were followed until either their next live births (parity $i + 1$) or to the study cutoff on April 30, 1970. The mortality experience of these women was taken as the number of child deaths occurring irrespective of age of child death up to the onset of the interval. Retrospective data from Pakistan were treated in a similar manner. All live births (parity i) occurring to Pakistani women from January 1, 1960 to December 31, 1968 were treated as the beginning of an interval. These intervals were followed until the next live birth (parity $i + 1$) or to the study cutoff at the end of 1968. The mortality experience of each woman was obtained by computing the number of live births and the number of deaths among these births at the beginning of each interval.

Before proceeding further, it is important to recognize that the computed intervals in Pakistan differ from those of Bangladesh. From retrospective pregnancy histories, Pakistan birth intervals were obtained by following live births between 1960 and 1968 to either the next live birth or the time of interview. Thus, one Pakistani woman may have several intervals included in this analysis. In Bangladesh, on the other hand, *women* were followed from one live birth either to the next or to the study cutoff. One Bangladesh woman therefore may contribute only one interval to this analysis. This distinction is important because interval lengths may depend on the method of computation. In the classification of Wolfers, Pakistan findings reported here relate to birth-interval births while Bangladesh data relate to birth-interval women (Wolfers, 1968, 1969).

RESULTS

Because the relationship of mortality to fertility may vary between geocultural regions experiencing differing levels of mortality and reproductive performance, it seems worthwhile to begin by reviewing briefly the demographic setting of the two populations under study. Such a review is presented in Table 6.2, which shows selected fertility, mortality, and contraceptive usage measures for Pakistan and Bangladesh.

TABLE 6.2

Selected Fertility, Mortality, and Contraceptive Usage Rates in
Pakistan and Bangladesh Study Populations

Rates	Pakistan	Bangladesh
Fertility		
Crude birth rate[a]	52.0	45.7
Total fertility rate[b]	6.4	6.2
Mortality		
Crude death rate[a]	18.0	15.3
Infant mortality rate[c]	120.8	127.5
Childhood death rate[a] (age 1-4)	--	25.8
Contraceptive usage		
Ever use[d]	11.2	6.4[e]
Current use[d]	5.2	3.7[e]

[a]Per 1000 population.

[b]Births per woman.

[c]Per 1000 live births.

[d]Percentage of eligible women.

[e]National estimates (married women aged 15-44 years).

As the data indicate, these two nations had moderately high levels of fertility. The crude birth rates were 52 and 46 per 1000 for Pakistan and Bangladesh, respectively.[1] The total fertility rates were nearly identical, slightly over 6 live births per woman. These populations also had moderately high levels of mortality. The crude death rates were about 15 to 18 per 1000, and the infant mortality rates were above 120 per 1000 live births. The childhood (1–4 years) death rate in Bangladesh was about 26 per 1000.

The fertility and mortality indices of these two populations therefore were very similar. An average woman experienced about 6 live births over a reproductive lifetime. Of these births, about 12% died in infancy and another 10% between the ages of 1 and 4 years. Altogether, only slightly more than 75% of all live births survived the first five years of life.

Data in Table 6.2 also show that these two populations have been highly

[1] The Pakistan total fertility, infant mortality, and contraceptive use rates come from the Government of Pakistan, 1974. The crude birth and death rates are taken from Pakistan Institute of Development Economics, 1971. The Bangladesh data come from the following sources: Curlin and Hossain, 1976; and Sirageldin *et al.,* 1975.

resistant to fertility control efforts. Despite an intensive nationwide family planning program beginning in 1965, contraceptive usage rates in 1968–1969 were so low that these populations could be considered essentially noncontracepting societies. The prevalence of ever and current contraceptive use in Pakistan was only 11.2 and 5.2%, respectively (Government of Pakistan, 1974). The corresponding figures for Bangladesh were 6.4 and 3.7% (Sirageldin *et al.,* 1975). While an examination of the causes responsible for these low usage rates is beyond the scope of this chapter, it has been advanced that high levels of child mortality may have been one critical impediment to effective fertility control efforts. This hypothesis is the issue addressed in this chapter.

A common analytical method employed in several earlier studies has been to examine the cumulative fertility of women with and without child death experiences. Such a comparison is shown in Table 6.3. This table presents the average member of children ever born according to the age of the mother and the number of previous child deaths for the Pakistan and Bangladesh data separately. Within each age group, those with child death consistently demonstrated higher cumulative fertility, and the greater the number of deaths, the higher the fertility. This positive relationship holds within all age groups and within each set of national data. In all groups, the number of children ever born is higher in Bangladesh than in Pakistan. This is caused in part by the selection procedure employed with the Bangladesh data. The Bangladesh study population was

TABLE 6.3

Average Number of Children Ever Born by Age of Mother and Number of Child Deaths in Pakistan and Matlab thana, Bangladesh

Number of child deaths	Age of mother					
	15-24	25-29	30-34	35-39	40-49	All
Pakistan						
0	1.1	2.8	4.0	4.5	4.7	2.4
1	2.4	3.9	5.2	5.5	6.1	4.5
2	3.6	4.8	6.0	7.2	7.0	6.2
3+	4.4	6.0	6.8	8.4	8.9	7.9
Bangladesh						
0	1.8	3.6	4.9	5.7	5.6	2.6
1	3.3	5.0	5.9	6.6	7.2	4.7
2	4.6	5.9	7.1	7.6	8.6	6.2
3+	6.3	7.4	8.6	9.4	10.4	8.3

disproportionately weighted toward higher than average fecundity since only those women producing a live birth in 1966–1967 were included, rather than a sample representative of all currently married women, as was the case in Pakistan.

Several researchers utilizing data and methodological treatments similar to those presented in Table 6.3 have concluded that the observed positive relationship validated the child survival hypothesis (Hassan, 1966; Wyon and Gordon, 1972; Harrington, 1971). But there are clearly insufficient grounds for such a conclusion. First, the influence of fertility on mortality has not been eliminated. More children ever born means, obviously, a larger number of potential child losses and excessively high fertility. Brief birth intervals could also cause high mortality. Second, while mortality experience may lead to higher cumulative fertility, the cause could be biological and not behavioral. In universally breastfeeding societies, early child death shortens lactational amenorrhea, thereby exposing a woman to the risk of earlier pregnancy than she would experience if the child survived. Thus, one is unable to attribute the observed effects to behavioral differentials alone.

Some of these problems may be reduced by examining subsequent fertility rather than cumulative fertility. One useful measure of subsequent fertility is the average length of time required between successive live births. Table 6.4 shows the median birth interval required to progress from parities (i) to $(i + 1)$ among Pakistani women, grouped according to parity and child mortality experience. These median values were obtained by life table procedures. As the data suggest, the interval between live births subsumes an average of about three years. With several minor exceptions, the median time between live births increases with parity. This pattern is

TABLE 6.4

Median Birth Interval between Parities (i) and $(i + 1)$ according to Parity and Previous Child Death Experience in Pakistan

Parity (i)	Median interval in months		Difference
	No child death	Child death	
1	36.6	31.4	5.2
2	36.0	34.1	1.9
3	37.3	35.5	1.8
4	38.9	34.5	4.4
5	38.5	37.8	0.7
6	39.7	38.8	0.9
7	41.0	39.7	1.3

expected, given the known effects of age and parity on reproductive performance. At the same parity, however, median intervals were briefer for women with child mortality experience. This relationship holds at all parities and is highly significant statistically.

The relationship also holds when the Bangladesh data are examined in a similar manner. Table 6.5 displays mean birth intervals between parities (i) and $(i + 1)$ of Bangalee women, grouped according to parity and the number of living children out of the first $(i - 1)$ births. It is important to note that the birth intervals shown in Table 6.5 are mean intervals; that is, they are the average of only closed intervals, including only women who produced a second live birth before the end of the observation period. Median intervals computed by the life table technique substantiate the

TABLE 6.5

Mean Birth Interval between Parities (i) and $(i + 1)$ According to Parity and Number of Living Children for Women Producing Births in 1966-1967 in Matlab thana, Bangladesh

Parity $(i - 1)$	Living children among parity $(i - 1)$	Mean interval (months)
1	0	19.6
	1	29.6
2	0	19.6
	1	28.4
	2	30.5
3	0-1	25.8
	2	29.3
	3	30.0
4	0-2	27.8
	3	28.4
	4	30.5
5	0-2	26.4
	3	29.2
	4	30.7
	5	29.9
6+	0-2	23.5
	3	29.6
	4	29.7
	5	30.0
	6+	30.2

relationship shown in this table, but they are not presented for the sake of economy.

Paralleling the findings among Pakistani women, the data in Table 6.5 show that within each parity group those Bangalee women with fewer living children (higher previous child loss) experienced briefer mean intervals when progressing from parity (i) to $(i + 1)$. Therefore these data also suggest a positive relationship between child death experience and subsequent fertility.

The difficulty with the type of analysis represented in Tables 6.4 and 6.5 is that the dependent variable (subsequent fertility) may interact with the independent variable (previous child loss) biologically as well as behaviorally to produce a positive relationship.[2] Any infant deaths of the parity (i) birth, as discussed previously, should result in briefer birth intervals between parities (i) and $(i + 1)$ among breastfeeding women. This type of bias is obviously present in Table 6.4. It is somewhat less troublesome in Table 6.5 because we consider fertility differences only according to the number of child deaths prior to the last birth. But even here the bias is not completely controlled, because the incidence of child mortality is probably highly correlated over the course of a woman's reproductive life. Several competent studies have shown that one of the best predictors of infant mortality is the survivorship history of infants of the same mother (Stoeckel and Chowdhury, 1972; Heady *et al.*, 1955). For reasons that are not entirely clear, some women are successful childbearers and others are not. It would be expected therefore that those women with high levels of previous child loss would also have more child deaths of parity (i) births. Disproportionately more parity (i) deaths in the child mortality groups would be expected to result biologically in briefer birth intervals. This then, rather than a child replacement motivational response, could account for the observed differentials of fertility.

This biological source of bias can be substantially reduced by comparing women with different experience of child loss but the same experience for the ith child. Table 6.6 presents the median birth interval of Pakistani women from parities (i) to $(i + 1)$, but all intervals where there is death of the parity (i) birth are excluded. Whatever differences remain in observed interbirth intervals can plausibly be attributed to behavioral effects. It is clear from a comparison of Tables 6.6 and 6.4 that the differences in median birth intervals between women with child death experience and those without has essentially disappeared when the outcome of the last

[2] Rutstein (1974) used multivariate analysis to examine the effect of child mortality on subsequent fertility. Fertility over a two year period in between two sample surveys was examined, according to previous child mortality experience. Unfortunately, interactions as described here between dependent and independent variables were not entirely controlled.

TABLE 6.6

Median Birth Interval between Parities (*i*) and (*i* + 1) according to
Parity and Previous Child Death Experience in Pakistan

| Parity (*i*) | Median interval in months | | Difference |
	No child death	Child death	
2	36.0	35.3	0.7
3	37.3	36.0	1.4
4	38.9	34.9	4.0
5	38.5	38.1	0.4
6	39.7	39.9	-0.2
7	41.0	41.2	-0.2

[a]Excludes women with parity (*i*) child death.

birth is controlled. Women with previous child loss in parities 2 through 5 have slightly briefer median intervals (higher fertility), but the relationship is reversed in the last two parity groups. Statistically, the differences are not significant.

Similar results were found among Bangalee women. The construction of Table 6.7 is identical to that of Table 6.5 except that mean intervals were separated according to survivorship of parity *(i)* births. Intervals with infant deaths of parity *(i)* births are displayed separately. When intervals with infant deaths (biological effects) are excluded, no behavioral effect whatsoever is observed. Within each parity group, there was no systematic difference in mean birth intervals between women with varying numbers of living children.

The absence of a child replacement motivation response on subsequent fertility is also suggested by Table 6.8 where median rather than mean birth intervals are computed for Bangalee women. Again, within each parity group, there is no difference in median birth intervals between women with varying levels of child death experience. The group that may be an exception is parity 6 or more, where median birth intervals decreased with fewer numbers of living children. One is tempted to conclude that these differences are attributable to behavioral effects, confirming the child survival hypothesis. Two limitations, unfortunately, qualify this conclusion. First, the median value of those with six or more living children was not computed directly. Because of the brevity of the observation period, this figure is an extrapolated value. Second and more important, there is an age distributional bias in the data which would tend to produce the relationship shown among women of parity 6 or more. Women at parity 6 or more with only two or three living children had at least three or

TABLE 6.7

Mean Birth Interval between Parities (*i*) and (*i* + 1) According to Parity, Number of Living Children, and Survivorship of Parity (*i*) Birth during Infancy for Women Producing Births in 1966-1967 in Matlab thana, Bangladesh

Parity (*i* − 1)	Living children among parity (*i* − 1)	Mean interval in months between parities (*i*) and (*i* + 1)			
		Infant death of parity (*i*)		No infant death of parity (*i*)	
		Months	*N*	Months	*N*
0-1	0-1	19.5	100	25.0	947
2-3	0-1	20.5	31	30.4	241
	2-3	20.1	40	29.9	552
4-5	0-1	-	1	29.6	20
	2-3	22.4	39	30.9	350
	4-5	22.0	30	30.1	269
6+	0-1	-	1	-	4
	2-3	20.8	18	29.5	96
	4-5	18.5	34	30.0	263
	6+	20.5	15	29.0	129
All		20.3	309	27.8	2871

Note: Intervals based on fewer than 15 observations are not computed.

TABLE 6.8

Median Birth Interval between Parities (*i*) and (*i* + 1) According to Parity, Number of Living Children, and Survivorship of Parity (*i*) Birth during Infancy for Women Producing Births in 1966-1967 in Matlab thana, Bangladesh

| Parity (*i* − 1) | Living children among parity (*i* − 1) | Median interval in months between parities (*i*) and (*i* + 1) | | | | Difference (Months) |
| | | Infant death of parity (*i*) | | No infant death of parity (*i*) | | |
		Months	N	Months	N	
0-1	0-1	21.6	162	36.6	1434	13.0
2-3	0-1	21.5	36	34.3	341	12.8
	2-3	24.0	55	34.4	849	10.4
4-5	0-1	--	3	37.6	39	--
	2-3	22.5	49	35.9	563	13.4
	4-5	26.5	41	36.4	468	9.9
6+	0-1	--	1	--	9	--
	2-3	25.0	27	41.1	191	16.1
	4-5	30.0	61	41.9	544	11.9
	6+	27.5	29	44.2	334	16.7
All		24.1	464	37.2	4772	13.1

Note: Intervals based on fewer than 15 observations are not computed.

*a*Extrapolated value.

four previous child deaths. At each death, these women would be expected to progress to the next parity faster than women without such deaths. Thus, women with this ratio of parity to living children are expected to be more youthful than their counterparts with more living children.[3] Natural fecundity of younger women is higher than that of older women, and differences in age composition could result in the observed differences in median subsequent birth intervals. An analysis of the age of women at parity 6 or more showed this to be precisely the case. The average age of women with three or fewer living children in this parity group was 30.8 years, nearly 5 years less than the average age of women with six or more living children (35.2 years).

Even accepting that a small behavioral effect may exist among women at parity 6 or more, the overall patterns of birth intervals in Tables 6.6, 6.7, and 6.8 are fairly conclusive. With biological effects adequately controlled, very few if any behavioral effects are detectable. In the sociocultural context of these two South Asian societies at moderately high levels of fertility and mortality, there is no evidence that child death experience generates a child replacement motivational response. If attitudinal or behavioral modifications do occur, they are not sufficiently strong to be reflected by actual reproductive performance.

It is clear that biological effects are much more powerful than behavioral effects in rural Bangladesh. The median birth interval for all Bangalee women whose parity *(i)* birth died during infancy was 24.1 months. The corresponding interval for women without infant mortality was 37.2 months. Thus, a difference of 13.1 months is attributable to the biological effects of infant death, interruption of lactation, and earlier onset of postpartum ovulation and susceptibility to conception. Behavioral effects, on the other hand, caused at the extreme a difference of only 3.1 months (Bangalee women at parity 6 or more).

The difference of 13.1 months attributable to infant mortality is consistent with previous studies on birth interval components in the rural population of Matlab, Bangladesh (Chen *et al.*, 1974). The median length of postpartum amenorrhea with a surviving breastfed child was reported to be about 17 months. Neonatal deaths abbreviated this period to only 2 months, and postneonatal infant deaths to about 6 months. With approxi-

---

[3] This same bias would apply to studies using the parity progression ratio to measure the behavioral effect of child mortality experience. Women in noncontracepting societies at parity (i) but with varying experiences of child mortality would be expected to differ in age composition. Those with child death experience would be expected to be younger than those without such experiences. With exposure to conception at a younger age and for a potentially longer period of time, women in the former category would have a higher likelihood of progressing to the next parity (i + 1) as compared to women of the latter group.

mately 60% of all infant deaths occurring in the neonatal period and virtually universal breastfeeding of all surviving children, the observed difference of 13.1 months in this study fits precisely with data reported earlier
on the length of postpartum sterility in Matlab thana.

DISCUSSION

Several qualifications to the findings reported here deserve comment.
First, the relationship between child mortality and fertility, as noted in the
introduction, is bidirectional. Mortality influences fertility but in turn is
also affected by it. Thus, while we have attempted to isolate and quantify
one direction of this relationship, mutual interactions are possible and
have not been excluded entirely. Second, not all potential behavioral effects are assessed. The child replacement response could operate primarily at the macrolevel, profoundly influencing a community's overall norms
and practices regarding childbearing and child raising. It is possible that
the magnitude of macroeffects is sufficiently powerful to obscure fertility
variations attributable to child death within a community. Third, the exclusion of fetal wastage information may lead to bias. If fetal wastages were
more common among women with child death experience, then the intervals between their live births would be disproportionately lengthened by
the time required for fetal losses. This would tend to operate empirically
against whatever behavioral effects were actually present. Available evidence suggests that the error introduced by this bias is probably not large.
Yerushalmy, for example, has shown that previous child death experience
is not associated with the subsequent risk of fetal wastage (Yerushalmy *et
al.*, 1956). Previous fetal wastage rather than child mortality is associated
with the probability of future fetal loss. Finally in our effort to isolate
biological effect, it is possible that some effects attributable to behavior
were reduced. In Tables 6.6, 6.7, and 6.8, women experiencing infant
deaths of parity *(i)* births were either excluded altogether (Table 6.6) or
separated (Tables 6.7 and 6.8). Yet, one could postulate that the child
replacement motivational response would be strongest for the birth immediately following a death. This initial and possibly more powerful response
is indirectly represented in this analysis in earlier tables, but it cannot be
distinguished from the biological mechanisms.

Despite these qualifications, the Pakistan and Bangladesh data presented in this Chapter make a convincing case against the importance of
the child replacement motivational response, particularly when the magnitude of the behavioral effects is compared to that of the biological effects. In Bangladesh, infant death shortened the median birth interval

from 37.2 to 24.1 months, a difference of 13.1 months. The largest behavioral response, ignoring the age problems discussed earlier, was only 3.1 months for parity 6 or more women. For all women combined, the behavioral response was essentially absent.

Thus any effect of mortality control programs on fertility in these populations probably operates through a biological mechanism. Better survivorship of infants, by facilitating lactation and prolonging the period of postpartum sterility, would lengthen the entire birth interval. The magnitude of this fertility-depressant effect can be crudely projected in the following manner. Given an infant mortality rate of 125 per 1000 and assuming the Bangladesh birth intervals shown in Table 6.8, the average birth interval in a population would be 35.6 months. This average is obtained by weighing the intervals of all women by the proportion of infant deaths and survivors. Keeping all other factors constant, an elimination of all infant deaths would lengthen this average interval by 1.6 months to 37.2 months. This is equivalent to reducing fertility by 4%, a modest effect by any standard.[4]

It is important to point out that this fertility-reducing effect of better infant survivorship is more complex when viewed in terms of population growth rates. While fertility would be reduced, survivorship, a central element of net reproduction, would be improved. From the persepctive of a population replacing itself into the next generation, reduced mortality of infants would have dual effects: a reduction of fertility but better survivorship of those infants who are born. Computation of these competing effects is straightforward. During 1966–1967, the gross reproduction rate in Matlab Bangladesh was 3.31 daughters per woman. Abridged life tables of current mortality schedules indicated that .7389 of female live births survived to 27.5 years, giving an approximate net reproduction rate of 2.45. With the complete elimination of infant deaths, the gross reproduction rate would decline to 3.17 (4% decline), but the proportion of women surviving to 27.5 years would increase to .8247, thereby resulting in a net reproduction rate of 2.61 (7% increase).

In essentially noncontracepting populations, such as those in South Asia, the common expectation that behavioral responses would be reflected by higher conception rates than normal among women at risk to pregnancy (or briefer birth intervals) may be too simplistic. Because contraceptive usage is essentially absent, regularly ovulating women in these societies already have high conception rates. Thus, even if women with child loss were to desire consciously to replace child loss and to act accordingly, it would be very difficult for them to achieve much faster

---

[4] These computations are similar to those suggested by Keyfitz, 1971.

rates of conception than normal women. The changes therefore would have to come from women without child loss who, having achieved their desired family size, would prolong their birth intervals by contraception. But such a response is unlikely if desired family size exceeds the biological maximum that can be produced. It is likely to occur only in transitional or industrialized societies where mortality levels are already low, where most women are already contracepting, and where the validity of the child survival hypothesis is less important for policy forumlation.

This conceptual framework assumes, perhaps too simplistically, that the motivational response is determined by gaps between desired and actual family size. It further assumes that women who attain their desired family size before completing their reproductive years would deliberately act to reduce their fertility by utilizing contraceptive methods that were readily available to them. But as Coale recently concluded from studies of historical populations, fertility control in a society may remain at low levels, even under circumstances where individuals perceive it to be to their advantage to have fewer children, unless fertility control is within the calculus of choice of individual couples and means to contracept are known and available to the population (Coale, 1973). Empirical studies from varying geocultural regions, at differing levels of fertility and mortality and with varying levels of contraceptive opportunities, therefore would be useful in any attempt to understand the effects of mortality on fertility. Even with these efforts, however, the conceptual and methodological barriers to a comprehensive and conclusive investigation of this relationship remain formidable.

SUMMARY

This chapter presents an empirical analysis of the effects, behavioral and biological, of child mortality experience on subsequent fertility in two Islamic South Asian nations. Data for the investigation come from retrospective pregnancy histories of 2910 married women interviewed in the Pakistan National Impact Survey (Government of Pakistan, 1974) and from longitudinal vital registration data (1966–1970) collected by the Cholera Research Laboratory for 5236 women residing in a rural area of Bangladesh. The aim of this study was to assess the importance of the child replacement motivational response to child death experience after biological effects have been controlled adequately.

A common approach employed previously has been to examine cumulative fertility according to child death experience. In Pakistan and Bangladesh, a consistently positive relationship was demonstrated between the number of children ever born and the number of child deaths. This method, however, does not exclude the inverse relationship, the influence of fertility on mortality, nor does it distinguish behavioral from biological effects Utilizing a measure of subsequent fertility, live-birth to live-birth intervals, the study further illustrates another common pitfall. Since the risk of infant death, which abbreviates birth intervals, is associated with the reproductive history of a mother, women with child mortality experience are more likely to experience briefer intervals because of the biological effect of infant death. Behavioral influences therefore may be observed by considering only those birth intervals with survivorship of the first birth of an interval.

With these limitations removed, very little, if any, behavioral influences were noted in the Pakistan and Bangladesh data. Median birth intervals in Pakistan varied from 35.3 to 41.2 months, increasing with parity. Within each parity group, no consistent difference was observed between women with previous child loss and those without. In Bangladesh the median birth interval for all women with a surviving infant was 37.2 months. This was shortened to 24.1 months by an infant death. When intervals with infant deaths were excluded, little or no behavioral influence was detected among women at the same parity but with varying levels of previous child loss.

Even without behavioral effects, elimination of infant mortality in Bangladesh would reduce fertility by prolonging the average period of postpartum sterility. The projected magnitude of the depressant effect in the Bangladesh setting, however, was only about 4%. This modest effect, moreover, was more than counterbalanced by the increased survivorship, resulting in an overall increase of net reproduction by 7% caused by better survivorship of infants.

APPENDIX

The appendix consists of the table on page 131.

Appendix: Life Table Computations of the Birth Interval in Years between Parities 1 and 2 Births among Pakistani Women with No Child Death Experience, 1960-1968

Number of years after the first childbirth (X)	Number who had first child at time x and were under observation at time x without having had the second child (O_x)	Number withdrawn observation from between time x and $X + 1$ (W_x)	Adjusted number at risk of second birth at time x (O'_x)	Number who had second child between time x and $X + 1$ (b_x)	Probability of having the second child between x and $X + 1$ ($1000q_x$)	Estimated number without second child by time x out of an initial 1000 who had first child at time 0 (l_x)
0	840	99	790.5	5	6.3	1000
1	736	66	703	79	112.4	993.7
2	591	58	562	233	414.6	882.0
3	300	40	280	164	585.7	516.3
4	96	14	89	45	505.6	213.9
5	37	6	34	15	441.2	105.8
6	16	3	14.5	4	275.9	59.1
7	9	4	7	0	0	42.8
8	5	4	3	1	333.3	42.8

REFERENCES

Adlakha, A. L.
  1970 A study of infant mortality in Turkey. Unpublished doctoral thesis, University of Michigan.
Chen, L. C., S. Ahmed, M. Gesche, and W. H. Mosley
  1974 "A prospective study of birth interval dynamics in rural Bangladesh." Population Studies 28:277–297.
Coale, A. J.
  1973 "The demographic transition." Pp. 53–71 in the Proceedings of the International Population Conference, Liege, 1973. International Union for the Scientific Study of Population.
Curlin, G. T., L. C. Chen, and B. Hossain
  1976 "The impact of the Bangladesh Independence War (1971) on births and deaths in a rural area of Bangladesh." Population Studies, in press.
Government of Pakistan, Population Planning Council
  1974 Pakistan National Impact Survey, 1968–1969.
Harrington, J. A.
  1971 "The effect of high infant and childhood mortality on fertility: The West African case." Concerned Demography 3:22–25.
Hassan, S. S.
  1966 Influence of child mortality on population growth. Unpublished doctoral thesis, Cornell University.
Heady, J. A., C. Daly, and J. N. Morris
  1955 "Social and biological factors in infant mortality." Lancet 1:396.
Heer, D. M. and H. Y. Wu
  1975 "The separate effects of individual child loss, perception of child survival, and community mortality level upon fertility and family planning in rural Taiwan with comparison data from Urban Morocco." Paper presented at the Seminar on Infant Mortality in Relation to the Level of Fertility, C.I.C.R.E.D. Bangkok, May 6–12.
Henry, L.
  1961 "Some data on natural fertility." Eugenics Quarterly 8:81–91.
Jalliffe, D. B.
  1968 Infant Nutrition in the Subtropics and Tropics. WHO Monograph No. 29. Geneva: World Health Organization.
Keyfitz, N. S.
  1971 Social Biology 18:109.
Moseley, W. H., A. K. M. A. Chowdhury, and K. M. A. Aziz
  1970 Demographic characteristics of a population laboratory in rural East Pakistan. Population Research, National Institute of Child Health and Human Development, September.
Nerlove, M. and P. T. Schultz
  1970 Love and Life between the Censuses: A Model of Family Planning Decision-making in Puerto Rico. Rand.
Nortman, D.
  1974 "Parental age as a factor in pregnancy outcome and child development." Reports on Population/Family Planning, No. 16. Population Council.
Omran, A. R.
  1971 The Health Theme in Family Planning. Monograph No. 16. Carolina Population Centre.

Pakistan Institute of Development Economics
  1971 Population Growth Experiment: Final Report of the Population Growth Estimation Experiment, 1962–1965. Dacca.
Perrin, E. B. and M. C. Sheps
  1964 "Human reproduction: A stochastic process." Biometrics 20:28–45.
Potter, R. G.
  1963 "Birth intervals: Structure and change." Population Studies 17:155–166.
Potter, R. G., M. L. New, J. B. Wyon, and J. E. Gordon
  1965a "Lactation and its effects upon birth intervals in eleven Punjab villages, India." Journal of Chronic Disease 18:1125–1140.
Potter, R. C., J. B. Wyon, M. Parker, and J. E. Gordon
  1965b "A case study of birth interval dynamics." Population Studies 19:81–96.
Rutstein, S. O.
  1974 "The influence of child mortality on fertility in Taiwan." Studies in Family Planning 5:182–188.
Schultz, P. T.
  1966 An Economic of family planning and fertility. Journal of Political Economy 77:153–180.
Sirageldin, I., M. Hossain, and M. Cain
  1975 "Family planning in Bangladesh: An empirical investigation." Bangladesh Development Studies 3(1):1–26.
Stoeckel, J. and A. K. M. A. Chowdhury
  1972a "Neonatal and postneonatal mortality in a rural area of Bangladesh." Population Studies 26:113–120.
Stoeckel, J., A. K. M. A. Chowdhury, and W. H. Mosley
  1972b "The effect of fecundity on fertility in rural East Pakistan." Social Biology 19:193–201.
Taylor, C. E. and M. F. Hall
  1967 Health, Population, and Economic development. Science 157:651–657.
Tietze, C.
  1961 "The effect of breastfeeding on the rate of conception." Proceedings of the International Population Conference, New York.
WHO Technical Report Series No. 442.
       Health Aspects of Family Planning. Geneva: World Health Organization.
Wolfers, D.
  1968 "Determinants of birth intervals and their means." Population Studies 22:253.
  1969 "The demographic effects of a contraceptive program." Population Studies 23:111.
Wray, J. D.
  1971 "Population pressure on families: Family size and child spacing." Chapter 11 in Rapid Population Growth. Princeton, N.J.: Johns Hopkins Press.
Wyon, J. B. and J. E. Gordon. The Khanna Study. Cambridge: Harvard University Press.
  1972
Yerushalmy, J., et al.
  1956 Longitudinal studies of pregnancy on the Island of Kauai, Territory of Hawaii: I. Analysis of previous reproductive history. American Journal of Obstetrics and Gynecology 71:87.

CHAPTER 7

Effects in Rural Taiwan and Urban Morocco: Combining Individual and Aggregate Data

David M. Heer
Hsin-ying Wu

HYPOTHESES AND QUESTIONS POSED

For several years a major debate has raged concerning the factors determining the success of family planning programs in less developed nations. One school of thought believes that success is largely dependent on the availability of appropriate contraceptives. A second school of thought is of the opinion that while the availability of appropriate contraceptives will prove highly valuable, this factor by itself will not be sufficient to reduce birth rates to desired levels. The latter group contends that persons in the less developed nations are still rationally motivated to have large families and will continue to have them until institutional changes occur that will change that motivation. Evidence for this viewpoint comes from recent findings concerning desired family size in many of the less developed nations. For example, in Taiwan, a nation generally considered to have a highly successful family-planning program, the average number of children desired is still about four (Finnigan and Sun, 1972).

Several social changes have been proposed to reduced motivation for high fertility. A larger study from which this chapter is taken focused on two such changes: (a) a reduction in the level of infant and child mortality, and (b) a reduction in the high preference for sons. In the present chapter, concern is confined to the first of these. More complete reports on the larger study are contained in Heer and Wu (1975) and Heer (1972).

The possible effect of infant and child mortality on fertility and family-planning behavior and attitudes can be subdivided into two components: *(a)* the effect of the community level of infant and child mortality and *(b)* the effect of the individual experience of child loss. Differences in the community level of infant and child mortality can plausibly affect the behavior and attitudes of both those married couples who lose a child and those who do not. When the level of infant and child mortality is high, all couples who never suffer the loss of a child may, nevertheless, fear such loss and decide to have additional children as insurance against the possibility that one or more of them may die in the future. The individual experience of child loss may also have important consequences for fertility behavior and attitudes. In comparison to the couples who have lost a child, those suffering child loss may logically *(a)* compensate exactly for the loss of their children, i.e., end up with the same number of living children as those who never lost a child, *(b)* undercompensate for their loss, i.e., end up with fewer living children than those who have not lost a child, or *(c)* overcompensate, i.e., end up with more living children than those couples never experiencing the loss of a child.

In short, when considering the impact of infant and child mortality upon fertility behavior and attitudes, we must consider four different categories of respondents: *(a)* respondents living in a high mortality community who have not experienced the loss of a child, *(b)* respondents living in a high mortality community who have experienced the loss of one or more children, *(c)* respondents living in a low mortality community who have not experienced the loss of a child, and *(d)* respondents living in a low mortality community who have lost one child or more.

Our study was purposefully designed so as to be able to secure respondents in each of these categories. Accordingly, we were able to test two separate hypotheses for our study population. The first of these is that a high level of infant and child mortality in the community would foster high fertility both among couples who lose a child and among those who do not. Our second hypothesis was that at any given level of infant and child mortality in the community, couples suffering the loss of a child would have at each parity level higher subsequent fertility, lower use of contraception, a larger number of additional children desired, and a higher ideal family size.

In preparing for the Taiwan study, we chose to select a locale where family-planning methods were available and birth control was practiced. We selected two sites differing as much as possible in their level of infant and child mortality (given the constraint that both sties had to be farily close to Taipei). We also planned for a large sample so that the number of cases of women who had experienced the loss of one or more children would be sufficient to make statistically precise statements. Finally, we were aware that we would need to have a statistical control for many other variables which might plausibly account for any observed relationship between the two variables.

Designing the study so that interviewing would take place in two sites differing maximally in their level of infant and child mortality provided the opportunity to separate out an areal effect from the effects of differences on the individual level. For example, it made it possible to discover, after adjusting for individual differences in educational attainment, economic status, and the experience of child loss, that respondents in the high mortality area had higher fertility than respondents in the low mortality area. Unfortunately, if this were the whole of our procedure, we would not be able to state that the remaining difference in fertility behavior by area was caused by the difference in the community level of infant and child mortality. A plausible alternative would be, for example, that the remaining fertility difference by area might be caused by the lower average literacy level of the high mortality area and the higher average literacy level of the low mortality area. To discover the specific effect of living in a high mortality area, we would have to interview substantial numbers of respondents in each of many different areas so that we had, for example, substantial numbers of respondents in high mortality, high literacy areas, low mortality, high literacy areas, and low mortality, high literacy areas. Such a survey was impossible given our budgetary constraints.

On the other hand, we could seek to measure the specific effect of the community level of infant and child mortality through another means. This was to measure, on an individual level, the perception of the probability of child survival. If the community level of infant and child survival was to have an influence upon fertility, it would presumably do so by affecting each couple's perception of the chances of child survival in that community. Hence, if we could show that the perception of child survival was related to actual child survival and that differences in perceptions of child survival were associated with differences in fertility behavior and attitudes, it would suggest that the community level of child survival did have an effect on fertility behavior and attitudes.

However, no one had as yet attempted to measure individual perceptions of the probabilities of child survival. Therefore, we could not be sure that we would be able to measure these perceptions reliably. Thus, several outcomes of our work were possible, each with its own consequences for the validity of our hypothesis. These were as follows:

1. There would be no areal differences in fertility behavior or attitudes after holding constant individual differences in educational attainment, socioeconomic status, individual experience of child loss, and other variables on the individual level other than perception of child survival. In this case, we would be able to reject the hypothesis that the community level of child survival was an important force affecting fertility behavior and attitudes.

2. After controlling for differences in all of the individual variables including the individual perception of child survival, there would be no areal differences in fertility behavior or attitudes; moreover, individual perception of child survival would be an important source of influence on fertility behavior and attitudes; and, furthermore, the individual perception would be closely related to the community level of infant and child mortality. In this case, we would have confirmed the hypothesis that the community level of child survival affected fertility.

3. There would be substantial areal differences in fertility behavior or attitudes after holding constant differences in all of the individual variables including the perception of child survival; however, individual perception of child survival could be measured only with a low degree of reliability and would not be substantially associated with fertility differences. In this case, we would not have compelling evidence that the community mortality level affected fertility; nevertheless, we would have grounds for belief that the community level of infant and child mortality might be an important factor in explaining differences in fertility.

Our procedure for testing whether the individual experience of child loss had an effect on fertility behavior and attitudes was much simpler than our procedure for testing whether the community level of child survival had such an effect. To test these hypotheses, we needed a large enough number of cases to obtain statistical precision, and we needed to hold constant those variables that might be associated with the experience of child loss and had been shown from previous studies to be importantly related to fertility behavior and attitudes.

The set of associations between early child death and the length of lactation on the one hand and between the length of lactation and the length of the subsequent birth interval on the other hand was one such factor that previous work had shown to be important. If a child dies soon after birth, a mother who has been breastfeeding soon ceases her lactation and the period of postpartum amenorrhea associated with lactation comes to an end. For this strictly biological reason, in a population in which prolonged breastfeeding is common, a woman experiencing the early loss of her baby will have a shorter interval to the next birth, other things being equal, than a woman who does not experience such a loss. Accordingly, in tabulations where the dependent variable was the voluntary fertility subsequent to a referenced birth, we controlled for the strictly biological effect of the association between child death in early births and the length of the interval between these births by controlling for the length of time between the interview and the referenced birth rather than between the interview and the first marriage. In addition, we controlled for the possibility that some women might be habitual short-term breastfeeders—who as a result might have both more deaths among their early births and shorter periods of postpartum amenorrhea after the referenced birth—by means of a control for the mean length of lactation after the referenced birth. We also held constant other variables which were shown in previous studies to have associations with fertility behavior and attitudes. These included the wife's age, educational attainment, birth control knowledge, labor-force status, and the husband's income.

SETTING FOR THE TAIWAN SURVEY, DETAILS OF THE DATA COLLECTION, AND CHARACTERISTICS OF THE RESPONDENTS

Setting for the Survey

Interviews were conducted in the low mortality community of Hsinchuang township and the high mortality community of Kungliao township. Both townships are located in Taipei county. It was originally contemplated that both sites would be rural townships. Because Hsinchuang had a considerably larger population than the original choice for the low mortality community and because it was officially classed as an urban township, it was decided that interviews there would be conducted only in areas outside the central town.

Much of Kungliao township is hilly or mountainous, and the large majority of the population lives directly on the seacoast or along the small river on which the town of Kungliao is located. Only a small portion of all land can be used for agriculture, and almost all of this is used for rice paddy. Because of the nature of the terrain, the roads within Kungliao are very poor. Hsinchuang township lies within the Taipei basin on the north side of the Tamshui River. Most of the township consists of flat alluvial land used for rice paddy. Although the township is situated a short distance north of the main railroad from Taipei to Kaohsiung, it is directly located on one of the main highways leading southwest from Taipei, and frequent buses travel to and from Taipei. Roads within the township are good although often crowded. The town of Hsinchuang is the site of both

Foojen University, a Roman Catholic Institution supported in large part with funds from West Germany, and the Taiwan Provincial Institute of Health.

Kungliao and Hsinchuang townships differed as much in almost every aspect of modernity as they did in infant and child mortality. The proportion of illiterates was lower in Hsinchuang, and the proportion of males engaged in agriculture or fishing was very much higher in Kungliao. Kungliao was quite unusual in the very high proportion of all males engaged in fishing. In 1966, the last year for which data were available, 42.1% of all employed males were fishermen. Fishing is done in small boats without the aid of modern equipment. Although the proportion of males engaged in manufacturing in Kungliao was negligible, the proportion so engaged in Hsinchuang was considerably higher than the average for all of Taiwan. There are many new factories along the highway from Hsinchuang to Taipei. The establishment of these factories was a basic cause of the high population growth rate in Hsinchuang and the very high rate of net in-migration.

The proportion of women 15 years old and over employed in a nonagricultural activity differs substantially between the two townships. In Hsinchuang township, it is somewhat higher than the average for all of Taiwan, but in Kungliao it is distinctly lower.

The contrast in mortality between Hsinchuang and Kungliao was marked. The death rate for infants and young children during the five years preceding the interviews was, on the average, at least twice as high in Kungliao.

Finally, consider the variables related to fertility. In 1969, the crude birth rate was actually higher in Hsinchuang than in Kungliao. However, this was not because fertility was higher in Hsinchuang but because of differences in age composition. The total fertility rate per 1000 females, which is a pure measure unaffected by age composition, was 4400 in Hsinchuang and 6130 in Kungliao. Despite the difference in fertility between the two townships, successful family-planning programs in terms of IUD and pill acceptance rates existed in 1969 in both townships.

In summary, although the two communities were selected because they differed so much in their levels of infant and child mortality, it was impossible to attain wide disparity on this variable without also creating very large differences in all other aspects of modernization.

Details of the Data Collection

The study design was as follows. The household registration system in each township was used to transcribe all households in which there was an ever married female. In all such households, all ever married women were to be interviewed. In one-fifth of the households, currently married males, if present, were to be interviewed. Males were to be interviewed beginning with the third, eighth, thirteenth, eighteenth, etc. household in each lin (small subunit of a township). However, the study design with respect to males had to be abandoned, because of high rates of nonresponse, in favor of interviewing males in adjacent households as well.

Interviewing began late in October 1969 and was completed in November 1970. The number of completed interviews by township and by sex was as follows:

	Female	Male	Total
Kungliao	2677	501	3178
Hsinchuang	4137	863	5000
Total	6814	1364	8178

The percentage of eligibles who were successfully interviewed can be computed only for females. For Kungliao females, it was 77.4% and for Hsinchuang females, 78.8%.

A reinterview to determine reliability of response to the chief questionnaire items was a key component of the study design. The reinterview was begun in Kungliao township in November 1970 and in Hsinchuang township in January 1971.

General Characteristics of the Respondents

On the average, the respondents in Kungliao differed markedly from those in Hsinchuang. In Kungliao, average socioeconomic status was lower, desired family size higher, actual fertility higher, child survival less assured and perceived as being less assured, and the reliance on sons as the chief support in one's old age more pronounced.

However, the differences between the two townships should not obscure certain similarities. In both townships, the desired number of children was sufficiently high to guarantee a substantial rate of natural increase, and the preference for sons was quite pronounced. Although substantial proportions of respondents in both townships manifested their entire approval of birth control, the proportions actually practicing contraception were rather low.

RESULTS OF THE TAIWAN SURVEY

Dependent and Independent Variables

Let us now examine the results of three multiple classification analyses (MCA) (Andrews *et al.,* 1967) in which the dependent variables are respectively *(a)* the number of subsequent births among currently married women of third parity or higher with the third birth at least one year prior to the interview, *(b)* current or previous use of contraception among currently married females born in 1925 or later, and *(c)* additional number of children desired.

The main object of these analyses is to examine the apparent influence of what we shall henceforth call the principal independent variables: *(a)* the sex of the respondent's first three live births one year following the third live birth, *(b)* the number of survivors of the respondent's first three live births one year following the third live birth, *(c)* the number of sons born and whether or not they all survived, *(d)* the number of daughters born and whether or not they all survived, *(e)* the percentage of births who died before age 15, *(f)* the perception of child survival, *(g)* township—which serves as an imperfect proxy of the community level of child mortality.

It is obvious that the apparent effect of these variables upon the dependent variables cannot be examined without statistical control for other relevant variables. Among the most important of these control variables are elapsed reproductive interval since the third birth, age, the number of living sons, and the number of living daughters. The other control variables include the respondent's educational attainment (and newspaper readership), labor-force status, attitudinal preference for sons, educational aspirations for a nephew and for a niece, knowledge of birth control, mean length of breastfeeding (lactation for all live births beginning with the third), husband's occupation, and husband's income.

For women under age 45, the elapsed reproductive interval since the third birth was defined as the interval between the month and year of that birth and the month and year of the interview. For women 45 and over, the elapsed reproductive interval since the third birth was defined as the interval between the month and year of that birth and the month and year the woman reached age 45.

In discussing the results of these MCA tabulations, we refer to a result as statistically significant if the probability of occurrence is .05 or less in a two-tailed test. We perform two types of statistical test. One compares the adjusted coefficient for a particular category of an independent variable with the grand mean for all categories of that variable. A second type compares the adjusted coefficient for one particular category of an independent variable with the adjusted coefficient for a second particular category of that same independent variable. In computing the standard error for the first type of test, we make use of the formula devised by Kish and Frankel (Andrews *et al.*, 1967). In computing the standard error for the second type, we use the Kish and Frankel formula, except that we substitute $(n_1^{-1} + n_2^{-1})^{1/2}$ for $(n)^{1/2}$.

Number of Subsequent Births among Women of Third or Higher Parity

Table 7.1 contains the results of two MCA runs in which the dependent variable is the number of subsequent births among currently married women of third parity or higher for whom the third birth occurred at least one year prior to the interview. In run A, we use as a principal independent variable the number of survivors of the first three live births one year following the third live birth; in Run B we use the number and sex of survivors of the first three live births one year following the third live birth. In both runs we also use township, perception of child survival, and preference for sons as principal independent variables.

From Table 7.1, we see that the average number of subsequent children is 2.73 (among women for whom the median elapsed reproductive interval was 11.9 years). Run A, which shows the effect of child loss without regard to sex, reveals this variable to be of fair importance with a Beta of .05. If there are three survivors, the adjusted number of subsequent children is .052 less than average whereas when there are only two survivors, it is .233 greater than average. Thus after adjustment for the effect of other variables, respondents with only two survivors went on to have .285 more children than respondents for whom the first three live births survived. In other words, respondents losing one of their first three children had made up 28.5% of their loss by the time of interview. This result is rather precise since the 95% confidence limits are only plus or minus 11.8%. Results for women losing more than one child are much less reliable. Respondents in the sample losing two of their first three children made up only 6.4% of their loss (with confidence limits of plus or minus 14.0%), and respondents losing all of their first three made up only 3.2% of their loss (with the very wide confidence limits of ±31.7%).

In Run B we show the effect of the number and sex of survivors from the first three live births. When there have been no child deaths, there are, after adjustment, fewer subsequent births as the number of males among the first three births increases. Adjusted subsequent fertility after three surviving sons is significantly lower than fertility after three surviving

TABLE 7.1

Number of Subsequent Births among Currently Married Women of Third Parity or Higher with Third Birth at Least One Year Prior to the Interview. Taiwan Survey

	Run	
	A	B
Mean: 2.729		
Number of cases: 3898		
Standard deviations: 2.261		
Value of multiple r^2	.632	.633

Rank of each predictor in terms of size of β

	A	B
Elapsed reproductive interval since third birth[a]	.820	.820
Mean length of lactation of all live births beginning with the third[b]	.156	.154
Age[c]	.141	.139
Township	.078	.077
Educational attainment[d]	.076	.076
Number and sex of survivors of the first three live births at one year following the mother's third live birth	--	.062
Number of survivors of the first three live births one year following the mother's third live birth	.046	--
Preference for sons[e]	.040	.039
Husband's income[f]	.032	.032
Educational aspirations for nephew[g]	.031	.030
Perception of child survival	.028	.029
Labor-force status[h]	.027	.028
Husband's occupation[i]	.027	.027
Birth control knowledge[j]	.006	.005

	Deviation from grand mean	Adjusted coefficient in run		Number of cases
		A	B	
Township				
Kingliao	+0.588	+0.201	+0.199	1091
Hsinchuang	-0.450	-0.154	-0.152	2207
Number and sex of survivors of the first three live births at one year following the mother's third live birth				
3 sons	-0.372	--	-0.149	358

TABLE 7.1 *(Continued)*

	Deviation from grand mean	Adjusted coefficient in run		Number of Cases
		A	B	
3 daughters	-0.160	--	+0.163	357
2 sons, 1 daughter	-0.431	--	-0.142	1136
1 son, 2 daughters	-0.411	--	+0.002	1150
2 sons, 0 daughters	+1.130	--	+0.261	170
2 sons, 0 daughters	+1.065	--	+0.227	161
1 son, 1 daughter	+1.050	--	+0.219	294
1 son 0 daughters	+1.521	--	-0.039	44
1 daughter, 0 sons	+1.977	--	+0.167	51
No surviving children	+1.646	--	+0.048	8
N.A.	+1.768	--	+0.006	169
Number of survivors of the first three live births at one year following the mother's third live birth				
3 survivors	-0.384	-0.052	--	3001
2 survivors	+1.076	+0.233	--	625
1 survivor	+1.766	+0.075	--	95
0 survivors	+1.646	+0.044	--	8
N.A.	+1.768	+0.007	--	169
Perception of child survival				
Less than 85% survival	+0.677	+0.234	+0.242	239
85-94% survival	+0.269	-0.005	-0.001	1133
95% or more survival	-0.209	-0.025	-0.027	2415
N.A.	+0.343	+0.085	+0.075	111

[a] One to 2 years, each subsequent single year to 23 to 24 years, 24 or more, N.A.

[b] No lactation, less than 6 months, 6 to 11 months, 12 to 17 months, 18 months or more, N.A.

[c] Under 25, 25-29, 30-34, 35-39, 40-44, 45 and over.

[d] Less than primary school graduate, primary graduate but less than junior high graduate and never reads a newspaper, primary graduate but less than junior high graduate and reads a newspaper, junior high graduate or more, N.A.

[e] High, moderate, none.

[f] Less than NT$15,000, NT$15,000-NT$24,900, NT$25,000 and over, N.A.

[g] Low, medium, high, N.A.

[h] Never worked and would not work in future, worked but might work in future, previously worked, presently working, N.A.

[i] Fisherman; farmer; not in primary industry, worked for self or relative; not in primary industry, worked for nonrelative; not employed; N.A.

[j] Low, medium, high.

daughters. Furthermore, adjusted subsequent fertility after two surviving sons and one surviving daughter is significantly lower than fertility after one surviving son and two surviving daughters. Unfortunately, the sample—large as it is—does not contain enough cases to examine the effect of sex of surviving children on subsequent fertility if there have been one or more child deaths.

In both Run A and Run B of Table 7.1, respondents with a low perception of child survival go on to have about .24 more children after adjustment for other variables than those with a higher perception (the differences in both runs are statistically significant). However, because most respondents perceive 95% survival or greater, the predictor as a whole has only a small value of B (.03). Preference for sons also exerts a significant effect in the predicted direction. However, the variation in the adjusted coefficients between the categories of this predictor is relatively small.

Township of residence also has a significant effect on subsequent births. After adjustment for other variables, Kungliao respondents go on to have about .35 more births than those in Hsinchuang. If our measure of perception of child survival were completely reliable, we could state that the difference by township is attributable to some factor other than the community difference in child survival. However, the reinterview demonstrated that the measure of perception of child survival had very poor reliability. In a reinterview conducted approximately 12 months after the first interview, the questions on perception of child survival were repeated. The coefficient of correlation between test and retest for the question on number of survivors from 20 births was .290 (with an n of 5454) and that for the question on number of survivors from 100 births was .285 (with an n of 4800).

Of the control variables for Runs A and B in Table 7.1, only one deserves special mention—the mean length of lactation of all live births beginning with the third. In both runs this was the second most important predictor. Respondents with a very long mean length of lactation had substantially fewer subsequent births than other respondents. However, the largest number of subsequent births came from women with 6 to 11 months of lactation. Apparently, the women who did not breastfeed at all or whose mean duration of lactation was less than 6 months utilized contraceptive methods with greater frequency than other groups of the respondents.

Ever Use of Contraception

The three runs with respect to this dependent variable will not be presented in tabular form. The independent variables used are identical to those used for the runs shown in Table 7.2. The dependent variable was the proportion of currently married females born in 1925 or later who had ever used contraception. In each of the three runs, the value of multiple r^2 was .26. When one, two, or three sons had been born, respondents who did not have a son die were more likely to practice contraception, after adjustment for other variables. But the difference was only significant in the case where two sons had been born, since the small number of cases in the categories where one or more sons had died cause high sampling error. Analysis with respect to the number of daughters born and their survival again confronts heavy sampling errors caused by the small number of cases in the categories where one or more daughters died. With respect to the percentage of births who died before age 15, holding constant the number of living daughters and living sons and other relevant variables, there is a slight tendency for those who have had some children die to have a greater proportion ever using contraception than that for all respondents. However, the result is significant only for the category in which 25 to 49% of births died.

Contrary to hypothesis, a high perception of child survival is negatively related to current or previous contraceptive use, although the differences between categories are very small and are not significant. Preference for sons is associated negatively, as expected, with current or previous contraceptive practice. Although the difference in the adjusted coefficients is not large, the proportion ever using contraception is significantly greater in the no-preference category than in the high-preference category. The difference by township in previous or current contraceptive practice holding constant other variables is substantial and highly significant. The adjusted coefficient for Hsinchuang is almost 8 percentage points higher than the coefficient for Kungliao.

Additional Children Desired

Table 7.2 presents the results with respect to the additional number of children desired by currently married respondents with wife born in 1925 or later. Results are based on answers to the question "How many more children do you hope to have?" The values of multiple r^2 found in each of the three runs in this table—approximately .52 in each case—are higher than those observed for any of the other dependent variables examined.

The number of sons born and their survival, the variable featured in Run A, proves to be its most important variable, with a B of .48. At each number of sons born, the adjusted mean number of additional children desired is lower if all of the sons have survived than if some have died. When one, two, or three sons have been born, the results are particularly

TABLE 7.2

Additional Number of Children Desired among Currently Married
Respondents with Wife Born in 1925 or Later, Taiwan Survey

		Run	
	A	B	C

Mean: 0.660
Number of cases: 5543
Standard deviation: 1.079

	A	B	C
Value of multiple r^2	.518	.519	.523

Rank of each predictor in terms of size of β

	A	B	C
Number of wife's sons and their survival	.48	--	--
Number of living sons of wife	--	.48	.45
Number of living daughters of wife	.32	--	.30
Number of wife's daughters and their survival	--	.33	--
Wife's age[a]	.19	.19	.19
Township	.09	.09	.09
Percentage of wife's births dying before age 15	--	--	.08
Wife's labor-force status[b]	.08	.08	.08
Birth control knowledge[c]	.07	.08	.07
Sex	.07	.07	.07
Preference for sons[d]	.05	.05	.05
Husband's occupation[e]	.04	.05	.05
Educational attainment[f]	.04	.03	.03
Educational aspirations for nephew[g]	.02	--	.02
Husband's income[h]	.02	.02	.02
Perception of child survival	.02	.02	.02
Educational aspirations for niece[i]	--	.01	--

	Deviation from grand mean	Adjusted coefficient in run			Number of cases
		A	B	C	
Township					
Kingliao	-0.008	+0.141	+0.138	+0.139	1934
Hsinchuang	+0.004	-0.074	-0.072	-0.073	3609
Sex					
Female	+0.026	-0.070	-0.073	-0.073	4619
Male	-0.030	+0.081	+0.085	+0.085	924
Wife's age					
Under 30	+0.730	+0.297	+0.292	+0.301	2236
30 and over	-0.331	-0.134	-0.131	-0.136	3175
N.A.	-0.517	-0.220	-0.218	-0.220	132
Number of wife's sons (Run A and to left of slash) or daughters (Run B and to right of slash) and their survival:					
None born	+1.231/+0.830	+1.030	+0.643	--	899/1113
1 born, dead before age 15	+0.925/+0.337	+0.885	+0.360	--	26/50
1 born, not dead before age 15	+0.274/+0.126	+0.198	+0.058	--	1485/1532

TABLE 7.2 *(Continued)*

	Deviation from grand mean	Adjusted Coefficient in run			Number of cases
		A	B	C	
2 born, one or more dead before age 15	+0.283/-0.282	+0.283	-0.123	--	71/91
2 born, neither dead before age 15	-0.394/-0.207	-0.319	-0.188	--	1374/1167
3 born, one or more dead before age 15	-0.458/-0.523	-0.294	-0.231	--	151/129
3 born, none dead before age 15	-0.509/-0.458	-0.455	-0.350	--	742/645
4 or more born, one or more dead before age 15	-0.607/-0.607	-0.415	-0.336	--	303/249
4 or more born, none dead before age 15	-0.625/-0.524	-0.508	-0.382	--	461/546
N.A.	0.457/-0.427	-0.470	-0.278	--	31/21
Number of living sons (Run B and to left of slash) or daughters (Run A and to right of slash) of wife:					
None	+1.216/+0.789	+0.616	+1.019	+0.941/+0.560	934/1178
One	+0.262/+0.105	+0.048	+0.192	+0.209/+0.068	1578/1025
Two	-0.403/-0.249	-0.194	-0.323	-0.306/-0.173	1549/1328
Three	-0.523/-0.477	-0.353	-0.445	-0.431/-0.342	897/765
Four or more	-0.631/-0.537	-0.360	-0.483	-0.481/-0.365	585/647
Percentages of wife's births dying before age 15					
No births	+2.074	--	--	+0.373	254
None died	-0.026	--	--	-0.013	4360
Fewer than 25% died before age 15	-0.561	--	--	+0.047	505
25-49% died before age 15	-0.408	--	--	-0.160	340
50% or more died before age 15	+0.867	--	--	-0.094	83
N.A.	-0.660	--	--	-1.748	1
Perception of child survival					
Less than 85% survival	-0.068	-0.050	-0.042	-0.046	339
85-94% survival	-0.020	-0.020	-0.018	-0.019	1616
95% or more survival	+0.008	+0.013	+0.111	+0.012	3474
N.A.	+0.294	+0.086	+0.087	+0.091	114

The categories of the control variables are the same as in Table 7.1 except the variable "Educational aspirations for niece" is added with categories high, medium, low, and not available.

strong, and all are statistically significant. For example, when two sons have been born, those who have lost one or more of them wish to have .60 more children on the average after adjusting for the impact of other variables than those who have not suffered such a loss.

The number of daughters born and their survival, featured in Run B, does not have an equal impact on the additional children desired. The value of Beta is only .33, in contrast to the value of .48 for the number of sons and their survival. For each number of daughters born, women who have lost one or more daughters desire more additional births, holding other variables constant, than women who have not. However, the difference is significant only when one daughter has been born.

Run C tests the effect of the percentage of births who died before age 15 holding constant the number of living sons and the number of living daughters. The differences in each category are small and for the most part not statistically significant. However, if 25 to 49% of the births died, the adjusted coefficient for mean number of additional children desired $(-.16)$ is less than zero at a statistically significant level.

The differences by township are quite considerable and highly significant. In all three runs, township is the fourth most important variable in terms of the size of Beta (.09 in all three runs), and the mean additional number of children desired in Kungliao after adjustment for the impact of the other variables was .14 greater than average and in Hsinchuang .07 less than average.

The adjusted coefficients for each category of perception of child survival were all small and were not significantly different from zero.

The Net Effect of Mortality Change on Natural Increase

If the level of infant and child mortality had no direct effect on fertility, a decline in mortality would obviously serve to accelerate the rate of natural increase. Conversely, it is possible that the net effect of mortality change upon natural increase might be to reduce the rate of natural increase. For this to be true, the fall in natality induced by mortality decline would have to be of greater magnitude than the decline in mortality itself.

We have hypothesized that a reduction in infant and child mortality would have two effects, a community effect and an individual effect. Let us consider first the degree to which our results confirm the effect of the community level of infant and child mortality upon subsequent fertility independent of the effect of individual child loss. We hypothesized that differences in the community level of infant and child mortality produced individual differences in perceptions of child survival and that these individual differences in perception caused differences in subsequent fertility.

According to our hypothesis, there should be no direct relation between the community level of infant mortality and subsequent fertility but only an indirect relationship mediated through variation in perceptions of child survival at the individual level. Nevertheless, our results indicate that township is a more important variable than perception of child survival in explaining subsequent fertility after either the second or the third birth. A major reason why the direct relation between township and subsequent fertility still exists after control for individual perceptions of child survival is probably the failure to achieve reliable measurement of the latter variable.

It would be incorrect, however, to assert that the true effect of the community level of infant and child mortality upon subsequent fertility in Taiwan is the sum of the township and the perception-of-child-survival effects. This is because the two townships differ on almost every other aspect of modernization in addition to differing in mortality level. For example, in 1969 the proportion of illiterate females 12 years old and over was 26.0% in Kungliao but only 10.5% in Hsinchuang. It is plausible to assume that this difference in literacy also affected subsequent fertility.

We cannot yet answer the very important question as to the effect of reduction of infant and child mortality on natural increase in Taiwan. If the community level of infant and child mortality had no effect upon subsequent fertility, it is probable that a reduction in infant and child mortality would lead to an acceleration of natural increase because on, the individual level, couples apparently do not fully compensate for child loss (our tabulations indicate that up to the time of the interview compensation was far from complete; it is likely, however, that if we were to follow all couples up to the end of their reproductive periods we would find that compensation was more nearly complete). Conversely, it is possible that a reduction in infant and child mortality could lead to a reduction in the rate of natural increase. The conditions under which this is likely are *(a)* that the observed adjusted township effect on fertility measured nothing more than the effect of the community level of infant and child mortality and *(b)* that age at marriage and the perception of child survival were both substantially influenced by the community level of infant and child mortality.

Finally, there is a fairly strong possibility that under the conditions existing in these Taiwanese townships a reduction in infant and child mortality, other things being equal, would have little or no effect on the rate of natural increase. This would seem to be the most plausible implication of our results. The women in Kungliao desire, on average, .355 more births than women in Hsinchuang, after controlling characteristics of individual women. Let us assume that half this township effect is a result of the differing mortality levels in these communities, or .178. Let us further assume that .285 of dying children are replaced (this is the average extent of replacement prior to interview if one of the first three children dies).

We estimate that the probability of a female birth surviving to age 29 is .94 in Hsinchuang and .894 in Kungliao.[1] Thus, the total fertility rate must be raised by approximately 5.1% in Kungliao as a result of its higher mortality in order to produce the same net reproduction rate as prevails in Hsingchuang. Assuming a base desired family size of four, the additional .178 children in Kungliao whom we assume to be attributable to community mortality differences represents 4.4% of the desired family size. Furthermore, women in Kungliao would replace an additional 4(.046) (.285) = .052 children as a result of their higher mortality, raising fertility an additional 1.3%. The replacement and community effects would thus combine to produce a fertility rate roughly 5.7% higher in Kungliao, just slightly more than the amount required to offset the effects of its higher mortality on the net reproduction rate.

RESULTS FROM URBAN MOROCCO

It was thought that it would be highly desirable to replicate the Taiwan results with results from already existing surveys from other nations. Accordingly, inquiry was made of the Roper Public Opinion Research Center concerning all of the KAP surveys in their possession that contained a complete reproductive history, including dates of child death, and had a sufficiently large number of cases to allow for a relatively low sampling error. A survey from urban Morocco was found to fit these criteria. The urban Morocco sample survey was carried out in October 1966 by the government of Morocco. An area-probability sample was obtained in nine different cities (Casablanca, Marrakech, Rabat, Sale, Fes, Meknes, Tetouan, Tangiers, and Oujda). Many of the results of this survey are reported in an article that appeared in *Studies in Family Planning* (Division of Statistics, Secretariat of State for Planning, Government of Morocco, 1970). Additional analysis of these data was conducted by Robert Repetto (1972) who investigated whether the sex composition of

[1] We estimate the probability of female survival to age 29 for each township on the basis of the average of the 1969 and 1970 death rates for children 1 to 4 years of age in each township. We choose not to make use of the infant mortality rate for this purpose because it is well known that many neonatal deaths in these townships are not recorded. In Hsinchuang the average of the 1969 and 1970 death rates for children 1 to 4 years of age was 2.11 and in Kungliao it was 5.27. A life table very closely corresponding to the death rate at ages 1 to 4 for Hsinchuang in these years is West model 21 and to the death rate for Kungliao in these years is West model 19 (Coale and Demeny, 1966). The probability of survival for females to age 29 according to West model 21 is .94, and according to West model 19, it is .894.

children had any effect upon fertility. He concluded that women having more sons tended to have a larger total number of live births. This finding was contrary to the expectation that strong preference for sons should lead to fewer live births among women having a high proportion of male babies.

Attention will now be turned to two runs of a multiple classification analysis made from a subsample of the Moroccan respondents consisting of currently married women under age 50 who had experienced three or more live births. In each run, the dependent variable was the number of live births subsequent to the third which took place up to the time of the interview. The principal independent variable of the first run was the number of the first three live births which survived either to age 10 or to the time of interview, whichever came first. The principal independent variable of the second run was the number and sex of the first three live births which survived either to age 10 or to the interview. Of the remaining independent variables used in each of these runs, the most important was a measure of marital duration within the reproductive period. This was operationalized for women under 45 as the number of years actually married and for women 45 to 49 as the number of years married minus the difference between the woman's age at interview and age 45. (This measure is thus not always identical to a measure which would have been preferable—the number of years married before age 45. However, for all women under 45 the measure is identical, and for most women 45 to 49 years of age the measure is also identical. The only exceptions are women 45 to 49 who were not married at some point after their forty-fifth birthdays but remarried prior to the interview. For these women, the measure actually used is an underestimate of the number of years married before age 45.) Additional control variables included in the two MCA runs are the respondent's own age, literacy, birthplace, work status, age at first marriage, number of times married, birth control knowledge, and perception of change in child mortality since childhood in addition to the literacy, occupation, income, and birthplace of her husband.

Before proceeding further, we examine in what respect the independent variables in the Morocco runs are equivalent to those in the Taiwan runs with the same dependent variable. First of all, in the Morocco runs we do not have a variable equivalent to the township variable of the Taiwan tabulations. It would have been possible to employ city of residence as such a variable only if data on infant and child mortality levels in these cities were available, but since such data were not available, this option was not utilized. Second, we do not have a variable for the Morocco tabulations exactly equivalent to the perceived level of child survival. As a substitute, we have the respondent's perception of change in the level of child mortality since her own childhood. Third, we do not have a measure of the length of lactation for births beyond the third. Fourth and most important, for Morocco we have measured the total number of years of marriage before age 45 rather than the total years between the third birth and the interview. This means that for Morocco we do not control for the fact that the length of postpartum amenorrhea is shorter after neonatal death for one the first three live births than it is after neonatal survival for one of those births. Hence for Morocco the total interval between third birth and interview (or age 45) is no doubt longer for women with a child death among the first three live births. As a result, although the Taiwan tabulations largely permit examination of the effect of child loss only upon voluntary decisions to delay or curb fertility, the Moroccan tabulations include the effect of child loss not only upon voluntary decisions but also upon the physiological capacity to produce another birth within a given time span.

The decision not to use the interval between the third birth and the interview for the Morocco analysis, as was done with the Taiwan data, was made because of the high proportion of women in Morocco who had been married more than once. Obviously, for women married more than once, the total interval between third birth and the interview might overestimate the length of time they were exposed to childbirth. Of all the female respondents in Taiwan, only 4% had been married more than once in contrast to 23% of the female Moroccan respondents under age 50. A possible means of assuring comparability between the Taiwan and Morocco surveys would have been additional tabulations for the Moroccan respondents restricted to women married only once in which the interval between third birth and the interview were entered. It is possible, however, that such tabulations could give biased results. This would occur if the death of a child led to divorce.

With all these caveats in mind, let us now consider the results of these two Moroccan runs, which are presented in Table 7.3.

Let us consider first the adjusted coefficients in Run A for the number of survivors of the first three live births. After adjustment for other variables, the number of subsequent births is .24 less than average if there have been no child deaths and .36 more than average if there has been one child death. Thus, up to the time of interview there has been a 60% compensation if one child died (with 95% confidence limits of plus or minus 19%). Compensation is less complete if two of the first three births have died. Here there is a 37% compensation (with 95% confidence limits of plus or minus 16%). If all of the first three live births have died, compensation is 59% of the loss (with 95% confidence limits of plus or minus 12%).

These results appear to show a greater influence of child loss upon subsequent fertility in urban Morocco than in rural Taiwan since, with respect to the latter survey, we estimated that compensation for one child lost was only 28% complete. However, as pointed out earlier, the Morocco tabulations are not comparable to those for Taiwan, and certain biases built into the procedures used in Morocco tend to inflate estimates of the extent of replacement of individual child loss. First of all, for Taiwan the results of the effect of individual child loss upon subsequent fertility are net of the effect of the community level of mortality but for Morocco they are not. Second, for Morocco we controlled only for the length of interval between date of first marriage and interview whereas for Taiwan we controlled for the length of time between third birth and interview. Among women of the same age who have experienced the same duration of marriage, those whose first three births occurred earlier in marriage, for whatever reason, would have had both a greater chance to

TABLE 7.3

Number of Subsequent Births among Currently Married Women of Third Parity or Higher, Urban Moroccan Survey

	Run	
	A	B
Mean: 2.704		
Number of cases: 1849		
Standard deviation: 2.189		
Value of multiple r^2	.339	.342
Rank of each predictor in terms of size of β		
Marital duration before age 45[a]	.503	.502
Number and sex of survivors to age 10 or to interview of the first three live births	--	.176
Number of times respondent married[b]	.172	.174
Number of survivors to age 10 or to interview of the first three live births	.162	--
Respondent's age[c]	.090	.092
Husband's birthplace[d]	.073	.075
Respondent's work status[e]	.067	.067
Respondent's age at marriage[f]	.062	.066
Respondent's birthplace[d]	.061	.061
Husband's income[g]	.044	.045
Husband's occupation[h]	.039	.036
Respondent's birth control knowledge[i]	..025	.026
Perceived change in child mortality since respondent's childhood	.017	.018
Respondent's literacy[j]	.011	.011
Husband's literacy[j]	.004	.003

TABLE 7.3 *(Continued)*

	Deviation from grand mean	Adjusted coefficient in run		Number of Cases
		A	B	
Number and sex of survivors to age 10 or to interview of the first three live births				
3 sons	-0.351	--	-0.165	164
3 daughters	-0.070	--	-0.110	153
2 sons, 1 daughter	-0.243	--	-0.125	427
1 son, 2 daughters	-0.430	--	-0.448	398
2 sons, 0 daughters	0.574	--	0.654	126
2 daughters, 0 sons	0.239	--	0.348	106
1 son, 1 daughter	0.332	--	0.215	247
1 son, 0 daughters	0.737	--	0.529	77
1 daughter, 0 sons	0.727	--	0.426	58
No surviving children	1.696	--	1.522	30
N.A.	0.216	--	-0.125	63
Number of survivors to age 10 or to interview of the first three live births				
3 survivors	-0.300	-0.242	--	1142
2 survivors	0.375	0.361	--	479
1 survivor	0.733	0.488	--	135
No survivors	1.696	1.519	--	30
N.A.	0.216	-0.122	--	63
Perceived change in child mortality since respondent's childhood				
Less now	0.020	0.027	0.026	1111
More now	0.027	-0.001	0.017	242
N.A.	-0.059	-0.060	-0.066	496

[a]Less than 5 years, each single year from 5 years to 29 years, 30 years or more, N.A.

[b]Once, twice, three or more times, N.A.

[c]Less than 25, 25-29, 30-34, 35-39, 40-44, 45-49, N.A.

[d]Same city, other big city, small city, village, outside Morocco, N.A.

[e]Usually works, works from time to time, doesn't work, N.A.

[f]Less than 13, 13-15, 16-17, 18 and over, N.A.

[g]Less than 99 dirhams, 100-199 dirhams, 200 or more dirhams, N.A.

[h]Professional or managerial, self-employed proprietor and other white-collar, nonagricultural manual, agricultural, N.A.

[i]No methods mentioned, one or more methods mentioned, N.A.

[j]Literate, illiterate, N.A.

experience child loss prior to interview and a greater exposure to the risk of pregnancy subsequent to the third live birth. Thus the procedure used for Morocco produces an upward bias in the estimated extent of replacement. An important reason why a control for duration of marriage only rather than duration of time since third birth produces bias is that among lactating women neonatal loss shortens the interval between successive births. The approximate effect of neonatal loss upon the interval between two successive births can be estimated from data on the effect of lactation on the birth interval. For Taiwanese women, Jain *et al.* (1970) estimated that with the cessation of lactation, which of course would occur in the event of a neonatal death, the average duration of postpartum amenorrhea is about 7 months shorter. Similar results for the Punjab in India have been reported by Potter *et al.* (1965). Assuming the length of the birth interval is 36 months, a neonatal death would therefore reduce the average length of the birth interval by 19%. Of course not all child deaths are neonatal. For the urban Moroccan women, of all live births resulting from the first pregnancy who died before age 10, 20.7% died before the end of the first month of life, 32.4% by 3 months of age, and 54.2% before the end of the first year. Similar proportions exist for the results of the second and third pregnancies. In summary, it is likely that the shorter durations of postpartum amenorrhea associated with early death among the first three live births are an important component of the observed greater subsequent fertility among urban Moroccan women experiencing child death.

Let us next consider the adjusted coefficients in run B, which is concerned with the impact of the number and sex of survivors of the first three live births. Subsequent fertility is slightly greater if three daughters survive rather than three sons, but the difference is not statistically significant. On the other hand, subsequent fertility is significantly greater (at the .01 level) if two sons and one daughter survive rather than one son and two daughters. Furthermore, subsequent fertility is significantly higher (at the .05 level) if two sons and no daughters survive than if two daughters and no sons survive. Thus, in general, the results presented here confirm those of Repetto that there is a tendency among the urban Morocco respondents for the total number of births to be positively associated with the number of sons. These results are in great contrast to those for Taiwan where subsequent fertility was greater the larger the number of daughters among the early births.

Finally, let us consider, for both Runs A and B, the results with respect to the question of perceived change in infant mortality since the respondent's own childhood. In both runs subsequent fertility is greater, but not significantly so, for women perceiving fewer child deaths now than a generation ago. This result is in apparent contradiction to the Taiwanese results with respect to perceived level of child survival at the present time.

Another noteworthy feature of these two Moroccan runs is the substantial inverse relation (statistically significant at the .01 level) between number of times married and subsequent fertility, after adjustment for other variables including duration of marriage. This rather surprising result might occur because of some lack of reliability in the data concerning marital duration or because women of low fecundity were likely to be divorced by their first husbands.

Finally, it is noteworthy that literacy appears to be a very weak predictor of subsequent fertility. Moreover, contrary to what one might expect, with other variables controlled, the respondent's illiteracy is associated (although not significantly so) with lower subsequent fertility.

In conclusion, it is obvious that we do not have an exact comparison of the Moroccan and the Taiwanese data with respect to the effect of individual child loss upon subsequent fertility. Nevertheless, even at the present stage of research, it can be definitely confirmed that in both Taiwan and Morocco the occurrence of child death among the first three births serves to raise later fertility.

ACKNOWLEDGMENT

The major portion of the funds for the Taiwan research were provided by contracts between the Office of Population of AID and Harvard University: AID/csd 2153 and AID/csd 2478. Supplementary funds were provided by a grant from the Population Council to the University of Southern California. Grants from the Population Council and from CICRED were employed to analyze the Moroccan data. The authors are grateful to Perry and Jennifer Link, Dr. John Williamson, Dr. Nancy Williamson, Dr. Margaret O'Brien, Ann Bowles, Jacqueline Lustgarten, Betty Hu, Richard Triplett, Fred Bookstein, and Margaret Bermingham for their contributions to the project at Harvard University. At National Taiwan University thanks are due Dr. K. P. Chen, then Director of the Institute of Public Health, and Hsiu-mèi Hsieh. We are also indebted to Charles Hubay, Jr., Dr. Frank Nelson, and Beth Olsen of the University of Southern California. Grateful acknowledgment is also due the late Dr. Harald Frederiksen of AID, the original contract monitor, and his successor, Dr. Timothy Sprehe.

REFERENCES

Andrews, Frank, James Morgan and John Sonquist
    1967   Multiple Classification Analysis. Ann Arbor: Institute for Social Research, University of Michigan.
Coale, Ansley J. and Paul Demeny
    1966   Regional Model Life Tables and Stable Populations New Jersey: Princeton University Press.

Division of Statistics, Secretariat of State for Planning, Government of Morocco
   1970   "Morocco: Family planning and an attitude survey in the urban areas." Studies in
          Family Planning 58:6–11.
Finnigan, Oliver and T. H. Sun
   1972   "Planning, starting and operating an educational incentives project." Studies in
          Family Planning 3:1–7.
Heer, David M.
   1972   Determinants of family planning attitudes and practices. (Unpublished final report
          for Contract Number AID/csd 2478 concluded with the Office of Population of the
          U.S. Agency for International Development.)
Heer, David M. and Hsin-ying Wu
   1975   "The effect of infant and child mortality and preference for sons upon fertility and
          family-planning behavior and attitudes in Taiwan." In John F. Kantner and Lee
          McCaffrey, (eds.), Population and Development in South East Asia. Mass:
          Lexington Books.
Jain, Anrudh K. and T. C. Hsu, Ronald Freedman and M. C. Chang
   1970   "Demographic aspects of lactation and postpartum amenorrhea." Demography
          7:255–71.
Potter, Robert G., Mary L. New, John B. Wyon, and John E. Gordon
   1965   "Applications of field studies to research on the physiology of human reproduction:
          Lactation and its effects upon birth intervals in eleven Punjab villages, India" In
          Mindel C. Sheps and Janne C. Ridley, (eds.), Public Health and Population
          Change. Pittsburgh: University of Pittsburgh Press.
Repetto, Robert
   1972   "Son preference and fertility behavior in developing countries." Studies in Family
          Planning 3:70–6.

CHAPTER 8

Fertility Response to Child Mortality: Microdata from Israel

Yoram Ben-Porath

THE ISSUE

The relationship between fertility and child mortality has occupied a central place in demographic research. The "theory of demographic transition" focuses attention on the timing of declines in fertility and child mortality and has naturally invited speculation concerning possible causal links between them.

Some explanations stress the physiological aspects of fertility. But it is natural and potentially fruitful to operate within a framework where preferences concerning family size are given a primary role. This paper deals

This is a revised version of a paper presented at the Population Policy Research Program Conference sponsored by the Ford and Rockefeller Foundations, Bellagio Study and Conference Center, Lake Como, Italy, May 2–5, 1975. The Israel Foundation Trustees have provided financial support. An early draft (financed by NSF grant G. S. 39865 X) was written at Harvard University. I am indebted to Gary Becker, Zvi Griliches, Simon Kuznets, and Julian Simon for helpful comments, to Celia Hanfling for programming, and to the Central Bureau of Statistics for the data. Appendix tables containing some more detailed results are included in Falk Institute Discussion Paper 758 bearing the same title. Reprinted by permission of the *Journal of Political Economy*, 1976, vol. 84, no. 4, pt. 2 © 1976 by The University of Chicago. All rights reserved.

with the effect of child mortality on fertility; child mortality may also affect age at marriage and other aspects of household structure which have a bearing on fertility but are not discussed here. More important, a complete interpretation of the child-mortality–fertility relationship should take account of the fact that child mortality may be an endogenous variable. The prevention of death via nutrition, mother care, and real expenditure on health is responsive to the level of income and relative prices: when the desired expenditure on children is large, the implications of mortality become more important. In this chapter, however, the endogeneity of child mortality is not discussed, and only the causation going from child mortality to fertility is analyzed.

Hoarding and Replacement

The effect of mortality on fertility can be broken into two parts: first, we can assume that the preferred family life cycle is not affected by child mortality and ask what effects of child mortality on fertility are implied by the attempt to attain the preferred family size. Second, we can take into account the possible effects of child mortality on the choice of family size or life cycle.

The desired or preferred family life cycle is the desired number of surviving children by age of parents, with specifications of the relevant characteristics such as sex, education, labor force participation, and earnings. Obviously, mortality raises the number of births necessary to achieve a given number of surviving children.

Let us distinguish between two types of reaction to child mortality: *hoarding* and *replacement*. Hoarding would be the response of fertility to *expected* mortality of offspring; replacement would be the response to experienced child mortality. This is similar to a distinction introduced by Schultz (1969). If the children die very young and the mother can have another child, the same life cycle can be approximated by replacement. Where the age profile of deaths is such that replacement can reconstitute the family life cycle, replacement is superior to hoarding as a reaction, since the latter involves deviations from what would be the optimum family life cycle in the absence of mortality. If preferences are such that people have a rigid target of a minimum number of survivors at a given phase in the life cycle, hoarding involves a large number of births and the existence of more children than necessary who have to be supported in other phases of the life cycle. Motivated by the old-age support argument, Heer and associates (Heer and Smith, 1968; May and Heer, 1968) explored the implications of various mortality tables for the goal of having at least one surviving son (with 95% probability) when the father is old, and showed that high rates of fertility are required for attaining such a goal. If children are replaced sequentially, fewer births are necessary.

The superiority of replacement is clear, but of course it is not always possible. The risks of mortality are often quite significant beyond infancy. Parents may be afraid of a possible loss of fecundity or some health hazard that will make late replacement impossible or undesirable. The reaction to mortality which is expected to come at a late phase of either the children's or the parents' life cycle may be partly in the form of hoarding.

Mortality Effects on Preferred Family Size and Life Cycle

Actual or expected death may also affect the optimum family life cycle and the desired number of children. That all the implications of increased mortality are absorbed by other activities and commodities (the general standard of living or children's education in particular) may be too strong an assumption, and it makes sense to consider the possibility that mortality, expected or experienced, also brings about a revision in the preferred number of surviving children.

Several studies by Schultz (1969, 1973, 1975; Schultz and DaVanzo, 1970) explore the association of infant mortality and fertility and indicate some of the relevant economic considerations. There are also an important study by O'Hara (1972) and discussions by Leibenstein (1957) and others (see Lorimer, 1967, and the discussion in Simon, 1974). A recent study by Rutstein (1974) takes an approach similar to the one taken here. What follows will reflect some of this earlier work and will rely heavily on a model developed by Ben-Porath and Welch (1972, 1976). Some related empirical work is contained in Ben-Porath (1976a, 1976b).

Should child mortality affect the desired number of children? O'Hara (1972) stresses the importance of the time profile and costs associated with children. Disregarding now the effect of the event itself, if benefits and costs were balanced period by period (on the margin) and if there were no difficulties in immediate replacement of children, there would be no clear reason for child mortality to affect the desired stream of child services. If most of the benefits and gratification derived from children precede expenditure, child mortality reduces the cost of child services. If expenditure (or discomfort) precedes the benefits, child services are more costly with child mortality. In terms of the complete family decision, these can be viewed as changes in the expected prices of children. If the case of early costs and late benefits is more prevalent, a decline in mortality will increase the desired family size; this will counterbalance the mechanical replacement relationship only if the demand for children is very elastic.

It should, however, be appropriate to take account of the fact that the price of children is not given. Expenditure on children is determined, at least in part, by the parents and may be affected by mortality. Lower mortality may make it worthwhile to invest in developing various traits in children (investment in human capital) and cause a shift from quantity to fewer, more educated children (see O'Hara 1972).

Take a simple model where

$$\max u[q(t, x)n, s] \tag{1}$$

subject to $\pi n x + s = y$, where t = indicator of survival, n = number of children, q = index of child quality, s = consumption of parents, y = full family income, x = inputs into children, and π = the price of one unit of x. Both optimum quality of children, q^*, and optimum expenditure on them, x^*, can be solved as a function of survival (t). The solution of (1) is (2) (see Ben-Porath, 1973b):

$$\eta_{nt} = -\eta_{q^*t} + \eta_{n\pi}(\eta_{x^*t} - \eta_{q^*t}). \tag{2}$$

The first term represents a technical relationship: as children survive longer, parents have more services, $(\eta_{q^*t} > 0)$ and need fewer children for a given volume of child services. The second term represents the effect of prices and expenditure. The term $\eta_{x^*t} - \eta_{q^*t}$ is equal to the elasticity with respect to survival of expenditure per unit of quality, $\eta_{(x^*/q^*)t}$. This term is likely to be positive and thus contribute a downward slant to the fertility–survival relationships via the negative price elasticity (see also O'Hara, 1972). If expenditure were independent of survival, we would have the simple expression $\eta_{nt} = -(1 + \eta_{n\pi})\eta_{q^*t}$, which, like the analogous case of augmenting technical change, indicates that fertility will be directly associated with mortality if the demand for children is inelastic.

This analysis would be appropriate if children were all purchased at one time. Further aspects become clear once we take into account the fact that most infant and child mortality occurs when the mother can still respond to the death of a child by having more children if whe wants to. We can think about this in the following terms:[1]

Compare two couples, A and B, equal in tastes and all the exogenous variables that determine desired family size, both sharing the same expectations with respect to mortality, and both having (e.g.) two children born. The difference is that B has lost one child. Assume now that A and B go on

---

[1] What follows is a straightforward adaptation to this problem of Ben-Porath and Welch (1972, 1976).

expecting the same survival rate for their remaining and future children. Couple B is worse off than couple A: it was hit in terms of children, while other activities were not disturbed. Adjustment means that B will try to restore some balance to its pattern of consumption—spreading the loss over various goods and services instead of losing it all in terms of children. If the demand for (surviving) children is income inelastic, B-like families will fully replace lost children; if the demand for children is somewhat responsive to income (or the degree of well-being), there will be only partial replacement. In other words, the extent to which B-like families respond to the loss of a child indicates something about the propensity to ''consume'' children out of income: absence of response would indicate a limited propensity, and full replacement would indicate zero income elasticity.

In the case just discussed, people are assumed to share the same expectations concerning future mortality irrespective of their own experience. But it may well be that both couples will modify their expectation concerning future survival as a result of their experience. This learning from experience would reflect the notion that, even if a group starts with a common prior probability of survival, when people realize that the risk of mortality differs between families they will use their own experience to learn or make inferences about how the true survival parameter relevant to their own children differs from the average for the population. This would fit a Bayesian paradigm with people starting with some prior probability which reflects the view held in the socially relevant environment; then, as they accumulate experience and as their own sample of children grows, they give greater weight to their own experience relative to the original prior probability. The inference from experience is the source of a substitution effect that is being added on to the income effect described earlier.

There are other considerations that this rudimentary model cannot handle explicitly. Pure risk aspects are not considered: in addition to the risks and experience of mortality, there are the risks and experience of unwanted births. Couples who find themselves with more surviving children than they want and are out of equilibrium will fail to replace a child who dies. This applies also to couples who choose a strategy of hoarding: obviously the strategies are substitutes, and if the stock of children was already planned on the expectation that some will die, the actual death of a child will not elicit a replacement response. Couples who fear (or choose a strategy that involves a high probability of) excessive births in the future may postpone replacement to the late phase in the childbearing period; except for such considerations, it is reasonable to assume that, since the demand for children is probably dated and since adding a new member to the family entails setup costs, people will try to replace children not too long after their death unless health or psychological problems interfere. To the extent that the demand for child services is somewhat reduced by child deaths, how is this reduction reflected in the length and timing of child service streams? What is the lag involved? These are questions that must be settled by empirical work.

Supply Considerations

Before turning to the evidence, I must remind the reader of the links between child mortality and fertility that do not derive from preferences with respect to family size. The link between breastfeeding and fertility has been widely discussed (see Potter, 1963; Jain, 1969; Jain *et al.,* 1970). In an environment where breastfeeding is practiced, there is a link between infant death and the mother's susceptibility to conception. In a context where (other) birth control devices are for some reason not available, child mortality will reduce the length of the interval between births and increase the number of births that a married woman will have during her fertile years. Thus, even this most mechanical explanation may have a behavioral element: It would work where breastfeeding is practiced and by what could be described as the elimination, by the death of an infant, of a (temporary) birth control device.

A somewhat more general hypothesis was offered by Knodel (1968), who pointed out that the presence of a newborn in the household is likely to be associated with exhaustion of the mother and with sleeping arrangements that reduce the frequency of intercourse and consequently fertility. This is a more behavioral explanation that would increase the variability of response.

A clear supply case is one where fecundity is an effective constraint, when the desired number of children exceeds the possible number. In such a case, child mortality will reduce replacement that may be bounded again by the physiological constraints but is not modified by revised demand.

THE EVIDENCE

In this paper the evidence is restricted to (retrospective) cross-section microdata. Thus, it is quite clear that the bulk of what has been described as hoarding cannot be caputred by comparing individuals. Expected mortality affects fertility differences among individuals if it is correlated (across individuals) with experienced mortality and the hoarding effect associated with learning is confounded with replacement. What microdata can indicate is whether replacement exists and how important it is. Two well-known problems in empirical work should be mentioned. First, mortality may be partly responsive to fertility—either as a direct corrective to excessive births or as an indirect consequence of the pressure of excess births on real income and thus on nutrition and health. Second, with microdata there is the ever-present possibility that left-out variables related to fecundity or to tastes affect both mortality and fertility, generating a spurious association between them.

The data to be considered here come from the special fertility section of a labor force survey held in 1971. This fertility questionnaire was a rider to the regular labor force survey sample and was administered to Jewish women up to age 64 who were married once and whose husbands were alive. The information used here is based on a list of all children born, giving their sex, month and year of birth, and whether they were still alive at the time of the survey (there is no information on the date of death). Thus it is not a history of pregnancies: Pregnancies terminated by abortion or stillbirths are not recorded at all.

The unit of observation is a birth. The first dependent variable to be considered is the stopping probability—the probability that a given birth is a last birth. The sample was too small to be restricted to women past childbearing age, but it was possible to confine the analysis to births of women age 35+ at the time of the survey.

Two important features of the Israeli scene are relevant here. First, the majority of the women are foreign born. Given the variety of countries from which they immigrated, their experienced fertility and mortality have a variance that is usually hard to observe in a single country. Also, when they immigrated, many of these women shifted from a milieu of extremely high child mortality, which they had either experienced for themselves or learned to expect, to a country with a very low rate of child mortality. This is, of course, just one element in the changing conditions and expectations that affect subsequent family formation.

The independent variables should in principle be of the following kinds: (*a*) Variables that determine the long-term desired family size. This is the role of the mother's years of schooling in our analysis (WEC). In one way or another, we control throughout for mother's place of birth, which in part reflects otherwise unexplained differences in desired family size. (*b*) Variables that describe the family's demographic situation at the time of the birth—mother's age (WAC), birth order (ORD), etc. (*c*) Variables that describe the family's economic position at the time of birth. Regrettably, this is totally missing. (*d*) Variables that are directly relevant to the main question being asked here. Dummy variables indicate whether a child has died (D) and whether the preceding birth (D-1) or any birth of a lower order (D-2+) died. As already noted, we have no information on the time of death of children. The procedure by which fertility is related to the death or survival of preceding births makes sense if indeed it is true that death cannot have occurred after the response is presumed to have taken place. Indeed, infant mortality is relatively high compared with mortality at subsequent ages; nevertheless, prior mortality is measured with error, and in principle this should bias the corresponding regression coefficients toward zero.

There are significant fertility differences by mother's continent of birth; the higher fertility of women born in Asia or Africa is reflected in their lower stopping probability at any birth order (see panel B of Table 8.3 below). There are also fairly large differences in child mortality by mother's continent of birth, with mothers born in Asia or Africa (AA) losing more children than those born in Europe or American (EA) or Israel (Is). Mortality is much higher for births that occurred abroad than for those that occurred in Israel. The proportion of boys who died is higher than that of girls (Table 8.1).

Estimates based on the vital statistics for 1960–1963 give infant

TABLE 8.1

Percentage of Children Who Died[a] by Place of Birth and Mother's Continent of Birth

Place of birth of Children	Mother's continent of birth			
	Total	Asia-Africa	Europe-America	Israel
Total	5.2	6.5	4.1	2.9 [b]
Born abroad	11.0	12.4	8.3	N.R.
Born in Israel	3.4	4.0	2.5	2.9
Males	6.1	7.2	5.4	3.1
Born abroad	12.3	13.5	10.1	N.R.
Born in Israel	4.1	4.5	3.6	3.1
Females	4.3	5.8	2.7	2.7
Born abroad	9.5	11.2	6.4	N.R.
Born in Israel	2.6	3.4	1.3	2.7

Source: This and subsequent tables are based on data of the Israel Central Bureau of Statistics Labor Force Survey (1971).

[a]Reported retrospectively in 1971.
[b]N.R. = Not relevant.

mortality for births in Israel at 26.4 per 1000 for AA women, 23.9 for EA, and 20.5 for Is (Peritz and Bialik, 1968; Schmelz, 1971). Data for the early 1950s suggest a similar rate for EA and a rate of close to 50 per 1000 for AA, which is declining fast (Kallner, 1958). These numbers are not inconsistent with the data in our sample for births in Israel.

The death rate for children born abroad can be compared with figures given in the 1961 Census of Population for children born abroad who died before the age of 5. The estimates were 23.5% for children of AA women and 11.2% for EA women, significantly higher than what we have in our sample. The difference may be partly due to the change in the age–education composition of foreign-born women between 1961 and 1971, but probably also to increasing omissions (response error).

We can now review the evidence in two ways—contingency tables and regression results. For a given birth order, the stopping probability is lower where one of the preceding births ended in death. The magnitude of this differential diminishes as one moves to higher birth orders (see particularly women from Asia-Africa in panel B of Table 8.2).

The lower panel of Table 8.2 presents the *relative* decline in stopping probability associated with one death. This can be thought of as the average degree of replacement that takes place. At orders 2 and 3, more than 80% of lost children are replaced among AA. At higher orders, there is a decline. The *relative* response is smaller among EA and Is; note that the initial level of STOP is higher in these groups. Similar patterns emerge when the probability of stopping at a given birth is related to the death (or survival) of that same birth. Among AA the effect of death is higher for births that took place in Israel than for births abroad. The relative effect is higher among AA women.

The treatment of each death as though it had occurred before the next birth, while in fact some deaths occurred later, imparts a downward bias to the effect of death on subsequent fertility. On the other hand, the fact that a birth is last in my data does not guarantee that it was the last in reality, although the restriction of the sample to women age 35 or older partly remedies this bias.

The difference in stopping probability associated with experienced mortality may be biased also because other variables which affect fertility and are correlated with mortality are not controlled. This is partly remedied in multiple regressions (Table 8.3). Because the dependent variable takes a value of zero or unity, ordinary least-square estimates can be misleading and logit estimates are presented. The derivatives of the stopping probability with respect to the death of last and preceding births are significant. They are much smaller (in absolute terms) for AA than for EA and Is women. However, when the derivatives are divided by the stopping

TABLE 8.2

Stopping Probability (x 100) by Birth Order, Number of Deceased
Children, and Mother's Continent of Birth[a]

Mother's continent of birth and number of deceased children	Birth order				
	2	3	4	5	6
A. Stopping Probability					
Asia-Africa (2267)					
0	14.4	24.0	28.3	27.2	32.1
	(492)	(387)	(272)	(184)	(131)
1	1.8	5.1	14.5	20.8	27.8
	(56)	(79)	(83)	(72)	(54)
2	0.0	5.3	0.0	8.3	39.3
	(10)	(19)	(22)	(24)	(28)
Europe-America (1155)					
0	62.5	70.4	59.1	46.2	42.9
	(664)	(240)	(66)	(26)	(14)
1	39.1	48.4	63.2	--	--
	(46)	(31)	(19)	--	--
Israel (566)					
0	30.0	51.7	48.6	47.1	38.9
	(223)	(149)	(70)	(34)	(18)
1		40.0	44.4	--	--
		(15)	(9)	--	--
B. Difference in stopping between women with 1 and 0 deaths					
Absolute difference (percentage points)					
Asia-Africa	12.6	18.9	13.8	6.4	4.3
Europe-America	23.4	22.0	-4.1	--	--
Israel	--	11.7	4.2	--	--
Relative difference (%)					
Asia-Africa	87.5	78.8	48.8	23.5	13.4
Europe-America	37.4	31.3	-6.9	--	--
Israel	--	22.6	8.6	--	--

[a]Women age 75 or older in 1971. Figures in parentheses are the number of observations (empty cells are those with fewer than 10 observations).

probabilities in each group, the difference between AA and EA disappears (see panel B of Table 8.3).

The pattern of the coefficient of D, D-1, and D-2+ shows a distributed response over birth orders. In the contingency table (Table 8.2), the effect

TABLE 8.3

Logit Estimates of Effects of Child Deaths on Stopping Probability[a]

	Woman's continent of birth		
	Asia–Africa	Europe–America	Israel
Number of observations	2278	1155	566
	A. Derivatives[b]		
D	-.033	-.121	-.096
	(1.3)	(2.6)	(1.3)
D-1	-.048	-.110	-.180
	(2.0)	(2.9)	(2.3)
D-2+	-.015	-.010	.092
	(0.9)	(0.3)	(1.5)
ORD	.040	-.005	.044
	(12.1)	(0.6)	(4.5)
WEC	.017	.008	.015
	(10.2)	(2.6)	(0.7)
$(WEC)^2$	-.000	-.000	.001
	(5.7)	(2.4)	(0.7)
BISR	.098	.038	N.R.[c]
	(6.3)	(1.3)	
NBAB	.002	-.052	N.R.
	(0.1)	(2.0)	
Likelihood ratio test	371.9	34.3	54.6
Degrees of freedom	8	8	6
$\bar{R}^2$	.225	.040	.124
	B. Means of variables used in regressions		
Proportion of last births (STOP)	.241	.615	.408
Proportion of children who died (D)	.081	.041	.041
Proportion of births in Israel (BISR)	.622	.757	1.000
Proportion of children with no siblings born abroad (NBAB)	.368	.594	N.R.
Mean years of schooling WEC	3.5	9.4	9.6
	(4.9)	(6.9)	(2.9)

[a]Women age 35 or older in 1971, birth order ≥ 2. Figures in paren theses are t-ratios in panel A and the standard deviation in panel B. The notation is as follows: D = dummy variable taking the value 1 if the child died; D-1 = dummy variable taking the value 1 if the child in immediately preceding birth died; D-2+ = dummy variable taking value 1 if child in any preceding birth (other than immediately preceding) died; ORD = birth order; WEC = woman's years of schooling; BISR - dummy variable taking the value 1 if the birth occurred in Israel; NBAB - dummy variable taking the value 1 if the birth was not preceded by any birth abroad.

[b]The derivative of the stopping probability with respect to variable x_i is $\delta p/\delta x_i = b_i \bar{p}(1 - \bar{p})$, where b_i is the logit coefficient and $\bar{p}$ is the mean stopping probability.

[c]N.R. indicates not relevant.

of mortality on stopping probability declined fairly steeply as birth order increased. When the stopping probability is regressed on mortality plus other variables in each birth order separately, the decline becomes less obvious.

Closed Intervals

The other dimension of fertility of interest here is the relationship between closed intervals and child mortality. There are several reasons why we can expect birth intervals to respond to child mortality. It is reasonable to think of a preferred family life cycle in terms of children's and parents' ages. The random element in births means of course that preferences can be only crudely approximated in reality. Still, the death of a child does not only elicit eventual replacement but calls for some attempt to have the new child not too long after the death. If the response to a death consisted only of bringing the whole timetable of subsequent births forward, we would expect the first interval following a death to be shorter than otherwise and all subsequent intervals to be unaffected. If the response to a child death were only to bring forward the date of the immediately following birth, the first interval following a death would be shorter, the second interval *longer* by the same amount, and subsequent intervals unaffected. If there is a distributed response over dates of subsequent births, it should be reflected in a shorter first interval and diminishingly longer subsequent intervals.

In a milieu of imperfect birth control, it is quite reasonable to assume that a desire to stop births would be reflected in longer mean intervals between births even if the demand for children were concerned only with completed size. Thus, with the appropriate ceteris paribus, one can expect movements in the intervals to be correlated with movements in the desired number of children. In addition, we have of course the mechanism that relates intervals to lactation and which may have an element independent of preferences with respect to family size (see Knodel, 1968; Jain, 1969).

By construction, the estimated intervals do not measure intervals between pregnancies. They are based on data for month and year of birth of children reported retrospectively in 1971. They are thus subject to large measurement error. The reporting error on dates is likely to be large, and the selection of sample by availability of response may be a source of bias.

The estimated mean closed interval is 33 months for AA women, 50 months for EA women, and 43 months for the Israeli born (panel C of Table 8.5). The mean interval in the three groups is smaller if the birth was preceded by the death of a child (Table 8.4). The decline in the interval for

TABLE 8.4

Closed Interval by Birth Order, Number of Deceased Children, and
Mother's Continent of Birth[a]

Mother's continent of birth and number of deceased children	Birth order				
	2	3	4	5	6

A. Closed interval

Asia-Africa					
0	29.1	37.9	37.7	34.0	30.5
	(17.0)	(23.8)	(28.5)	(22.6)	(22.5)
	(639)	(418)	(236)	(128)	(69)
1	19.0	25.8	27.2	32.8	25.8
	(7.3)	(16.7)	(26.7)	(18.6)	(14.2)
	(22)	(31)	(37)	(29)	(20)
Europe-America					
0	51.1	55.9	41.1	--	--
	(32.2)	(33.5)	(23.2)	--	--
	(711)	(238)	(65)	--	--
1	35.8	42.9	49.2	--	--
	(21.4)	(33.0)	(20.9)	--	--
	(30)	(21)	(11)		
Israel					
0	38.7	48.7	--	--	--
	(22.4)	(32.0)	--	--	--
	(357)	(183)	--	--	--
1	23.3	46.1	--	--	--
	(17.8)	(18.3)	--	--	--
	(10)	(9)			

B. Difference between 0 and 1 death

Asia-Africa	10.1	12.1	10.5	1.2	4.7
Europe-America	15.3	13.0	-8.1	--	--
Israel	15.4	2.6	--	--	--

[a]Woman with information on timing of births, in months (means).
Figures in parentheses are the standard deviation (first row) and the
number of observations (second row). Empty cells are those with fewer
than 10 observations.

second child (i.e., between first and second) is 10 (AA) to 15 (EA and Is)
months. When other variables are controlled in a regression framework, it
turns out that the relative, as well as the absolute, decline in the interval is
more pronounced among EA and Is women than among AA women (Table
8.5; age at birth and birth order are associated with longer intervals, and so
is schooling, among AA women).

TABLE 8.5

Two Regressions with Dependent-Variable Natural Logarithm of
Closed Interval[a]

	Woman's continent of birth		
	Asia–Africa	Europe–America	Israel
Number of observations	1767	1141	695
A. Regression I			
D-1	-.269	-.409	-.609
	(3.6)	(3.4)	(3.5)
D-2+	-.065	-.018	-.049
	(1.1)	(0.1)	(0.2)
BISR	.054	.157	N.R.[b]
	(1.4)	(2.8)	
ORD 3	.230	.057	.169
	(6.0)	(1.1)	(2.8)
ORD 4+	.160	-.274	.165
	(4.2)	(4.0)	(2.4)
WEC	.022	.004	-.000
	(5.0)	(0.6)	(0.0)
$(WEC)^2$	-.000	-.000	.000
	(3.1)	(0.8)	(0.2)
$\bar{R}^2$	.041	.032	.026
B. Regression II			
D-1	-.188	-.319	-.558
	(2.7)	(3.1)	(3.6)
D-2+	.044	.100	.033
	(0.5)	(0.9)	(0.2)
WAC	.053	.073	.077
	(16.2)	(20.0)	(13.5)
C. Means of Variables for birth order 2+			
Closed interval in months	32.8	50.1	42.7
	(22.0)	(32.0)	(27.0)
Mother's age at birth (WAC)	27.4	30.0	28.2
	(5.1)	(5.2)	(4.8)
Proportion of births preceded by death in preceding birth (D-1)	0.044	0.033	0.022

[a]Women with information on timing of births. ORD 3 and ORD 4+ are
dummy variables taking the value 1 for, respectively, birth orders 3 and
4+; WAC is woman's age at birth of child. Other symbols as in Table 8.3.
Figures in parentheses are *t*-ratios in panels A and B and the standard
deviation in panel C.

[b]N.R. indicates not relevant.

The analysis of intervals raises a number of problems. Couples with many children are more likely than couples with few children to have shorter intervals, on the one hand, and more experience of child deaths, on the other. This may create a spurious negative correlation between child -mortality and closed intervals and exaggerate the effect of prior mortality on the intervals. As a remedy for biases coming from couple-specific effects on intervals, deviations of the interval for each birth from the mean interval of all births of the same mother were used as a dependent variable. This indeed reduces the estimated effect of prior mortality on the intervals but does not wipe it out (see the three right-hand columns in Table 8.6).

For EA and Is women, the effect of prior mortality on intervals rises steeply with mother's age (and with birth order), but there is no such clear trend among AA women (sample size and lack of statistical significance blur the picture).

We can understand the change with age of the effect of mortality on fertility if we assume that the mortality to which older women react also occurred at a later age. If the preferred family size is small and the preferred childbearing period limited (and, correspondingly, family planning is fairly widespread), the response to child death is likely to become more urgent as the woman gets older because of the desire to avoid extending the childbearing and raising period. The expectation of declining fecundity is one element in the tendency to avoid late replacement. When fertility is very high and the childbearing period long and near the maximum, there is a constraint on possible reduction of intervals, because the intervals are short and closer to the minimum. It should also be noted that in families with many children there is greater likelihood that some of the children were not wanted or were born on the basis of expected mortality, and in such a case the death of a child will not call for replacement. These may be the reasons for the observed difference in response to child mortality over the life cycle between EA and Is women, the low-fertility groups, and AA, the high-fertility group.

Another issue of interest is the distribution of the effect of a given death on subsequent intervals. This is the reason for the distinction in the regression between D-1, indicating death in the immediately preceding birth, and D-2+, death in any earlier birth. Most of the coefficients of D-2+ are not statistically significant; they tend to be positive and smaller in absolute size than the generally negative coefficients of D-1. This would indicate that, when a death occurs and the next birth occurs earlier, subsequent births may not be shifted back by the full change in intervals, which is another way of saying that replacement is partial.

Finally, while we do not have a direct way of evaluating the importance of learning, we do have clear evidence that those who experience child

TABLE 8.6

Regression Coefficients of Closed Interval and Deviation of Interval on Past Survival[a]

Birth order and woman's age when birth occurred	Closed interval mother's continent of birth			Deviation interval mother's continent of birth		
	Asia-Africa	Europe-America	Israel	Asia-Africa	Europe-America	Israel
			Order 2+			
All women[b]						
D-1	-6.7 (2.7) (1767)	-15.5 (3.0) (1141)	-14.0 (2.0) (695)	-2.6 (1.4)	-5.8 (2.3)	-2.7 (0.6)
Women under 25[c]						
D-1	-5.2 (2.7) (710)	-7.7 (1.8) (240)	-8.9 (1.6) (226)	-1.0 (0.5)	-7.1 (1.7)	--
D-2+	--	6.9 (1.1)	12.6 (1.3)	3.5 (1.7)	5.8 (0.9)	23.4 (2.3)
Women 26-34[c]						
D-1	-1.0 (0.2) (876)	-9.0 (1.7) (674)	-13.6 (1.6) (391)	--	-2.1 (0.7)	-2.6 (0.4)
D-2+	-3.8 (1.4)	--	-8.0 (1.0)	--	2.5 (0.7)	--
Women 35+[c]						
D-1	-3.5 (0.3) (181)	-38.8 (2.2) (227)	-20.8 (0.7) (78)	--	-12.7 (1.4)	-14.9 (0.9)
D-2+	5.4 (0.8)	--	--	5.9 (1.3)	--	5.1 (4.1)

176

TABLE 8.6 *(Continued)*

Birth order and woman's age when birth occurred	Closed interval mother's continent of birth			Deviation interval mother's continent of birth		
	Asia-Africa	Europe-America	Israel	Asia-Africa	Europe-America	Israel
Order 3+						
All women[d]						
D-1	-4.0	-28.2	-17.0	-2.4	-24.2	-8.0
	(0.9)	(2.6)	(1.5)	(0.7)	(3.0)	(0.9)
	(898)	(337)	(320)			
D-2+	1.4	--	-2.9	2.6	2.5	4.5
	(0.5)		(0.4)	(1.3)	(0.5)	(0.7)

[a] In months for woman with information on timing of births. Notation is as in Tables 8.3 and 8.5. Figures in parentheses are t-ratios (first row) and number of observations (second row). The symbol -- indicates t < 0.5.

[b] Other independent variables are BISR, NBAB, WEC, (WEC)^2, ORD 3, and ORD 4+.

[c] Other independent variables as listed in preceding note, with the addition of WAC.

[d] Other independent variables as listed in second note, with the addition of WAC and excluding BISR.

mortality with first children are more likely to experience it in higher parities (not shown).

SUMMARY AND CONCLUSIONS

In the introductory discussion, I suggested several issues bearing on the analysis of the mortality–fertility relationship. The demand for children is not just a matter of completed family size; the children's ages at different stages of the family life cycle may also be an important dimension. The nature of the preferred life cycle reflects the motives for having children and the external conditions. We can explore the implications of mortality for fertility where the preferred life cycle is assumed to be independent of child mortality, or we can take into account the possibility that the preferred life cycle and family size depend on child mortality. I distinguish two types of response to child mortality, hoarding and replacement. Hoarding is the response to expected mortality, and replacement is the response to experienced or prior mortality. I note that there might be a learning process in a sequential framework when experienced mortality affects expected mortality.

The empirical work presented here focuses on microdata of retrospectively reported births of Israeli women. Tabular and regression analyses show that experienced mortality reduces the probability of stopping at a given birth (i.e., raises the number of births) and reduces the intervals between births.

The analysis was carried out separately for Jewish women born in Asia or Africa (AA), whose completed fertility is high, and women born in Europe or America (EA) or in Israel (Is), with lower fertility. The relative decline in stopping probability at low birth orders is higher for AA than for EA and Is in a crude comparison. Once other variables are controlled in a regression, the absolute effect is greater among EA and the relative effect is fairly similar. The response in intervals is higher among EA than among AA. It rises steeply with age among EA and Is and does not vary much by age among AA. These findings are tentative.

The findings indicate that replacement is a significant phenomenon and that it occurs fairly quickly; the age patterns of response can be reasonably interpreted. But the analysis of microdata for one group cannot bring out the factors or variables common to the individual units. Thus, if expected mortality is to a large extent shared by the couples in the sample, hoarding cannot be studied. It should also be noted that hoarding and replacement are substitutes; if families have learned to expect high mortality and respond to it by hoarding, fertility should not respond strongly to actual mortality.

This ties with a more important issue—one which is not, of course, confined to this area: aggregate time-series data indicate a fairly sluggish response of fertility to infant mortality (see Kuznets, 1973, 1974). How can this be reconciled with the findings of this and other studies based on microdata? Obviously, one would look for left-out variables that operate in one context and not in the other. One possibility would be that micro-response is largely spurious, reflecting left-out variables operating simultaneously on fertility and mortality. Alternatively, even if it is biased upward, the micro-response may provide a reasonable approximation to the partial effect of experienced child mortality on fertility, but in aggregate time series the trend in child mortality is associated with change in adult mortality affecting the parents' own fecund period and survival expectations, which may, respectively, increase the supply of and the demand for children, this in addition to aggregate developments other than mortality not captured in a cross section of individuals.[2] It would also be important to see whether in microdata the response to infant mortality differs from the response to other child mortality.

REFERENCES

Ben-Porath, Yoram
  1976a "Fertility in Israel: A Mini-Survey and Some New Findings." In A. Coale (Ed.) Economic Factors in Population Growth. New York: Macmillan.
Ben-Porath, Yoram
  1976b "Fertility and Child Mortality—Issues in The Demographic Transition of a Migrant Population." In R. H. Easterlin (Ed.) Population and Economic Change in Less Developed Countries (in preparation).
Ben-Porath, Yoram, and Welch, Finis
  1972 Chance, Child Traits, and Choice of Family Size. Publication no. R-1117-NIH/RF. Santa Monica, Calif.: RAND.
Ben-Porath, Yoram, and Welch, Finis
  1976 "Do Sex Preferences Really Matter?" Quarterly Journal of Economics 90 (May): 285–307.
Jain, A. K.
  1969 "Fecundability and Its Relation to Age in a Sample of Taiwanese Women." Population Studies 23 (1) March: 69–85.
Jain, A. K.; Hsu, T. C.; Freedman, Ronald; and Chang, M. C.
  1970 "Demographic Aspects of Lactation and Postpartum Amenorrhea." Demography 7 (2) May: 255–271.
Heer, David M., and Smith, Dean O.
  1968 "Mortality Levels, Desired Family Size and Population Increase." Demography 5 (1): 104–121.

[2] Some of these issues are pursued in conjunction with independent estimates of the mortality-fertility relationship in Ben-Porath (1976b).

Kallner, Gertrude
  1958   Perinatal and Maternal Mortality in Israel (1950–1954). Central Bureau of Statistics
         Special Series no. 75. Jerusalem: Central Bur. Statis.
Knodel, J.
  1968   "Infant Mortality and Fertility in Three Bavarian Villages: An Analysis of Family
         Histories from the 19th Century." Population Studies 12 (3) November: 297–318.
Kuznets, Simon
  1973   Population Trends and Modern Economic Growth. Economic Growth Center Dis-
         cussion Paper no. 191. New Haven, Conn.: Yale Univ.
Kuznets, Simon
  1974   Fertility Differentials between Less Developed and Developed Regions: Compo-
         nents and Implications. Economic Growth Center Discussion Paper no. 217. New
         Haven, Conn.: Yale Univ.
Leibenstein, Harvey
  1957   Economic Backwardness and Economic Growth. New York: Wiley.
Lorimer, Frank
  1967   "The Economics of Family Formation under Different Conditions." In World Popu-
         lation Conference 1965. Vol. 2. New York: United Nations.
May, D. J. and Heer, D. M.
  1968   "Son Survivorship Motivation and Family Size in India: A Compartor Simula-
         tion," Population Studies 22 (2) July: 199–210.
O'Hara, Donald J.
  1972   Changes in Mortality Levels and Family Decisions regarding Children. Publication
         no. R-914-RF. Santa Monica, Calif.: RAND.
Peritz, E., and Bialik, O.
  1968   "Infant Mortality in the Jewish Population of Israel." Israel J. Medical Sci. 4 (5).
Potter, Robert G., Jr.
  1963   "Birth Intervals: Structure and Change." Population Studies 17 (1) November:
         155–166.
Rutstein, Shea Oscar
  1974   "The Influence of Child Mortality on Fertility in Taiwan." Studies in Family Plan-
         ning 5 (6) June: 182–188.
Schmelz, U. O.
  1971   Infant and Early Childhood Mortality among the Jews of the Diaspora. Jerusalem:
         Inst. Contemporary Jewry, Hebrew Univ.
Schoenberg, Erika, and Douglas, Paul
  1937   "Studies in the Supply Curve of Labor." J.P.E. 45 (1) February: 45–79.
Schultz, T. Paul
  1969   "An Economic Model of Family Planning and Fertility." J.P.E. 77 (2) March/April:
         153–180.
Schultz, T. Paul
  1973   "Explanation of Birth Rate Changes over Space and Time: A Study of Taiwan."
         J.P.E. 81 (2) Part 2 (March/April): S238–S274.
Schultz, T. Paul
  1975   "Interrelationships between Mortality and Fertility." Dratt. Resources for the
         Future.
Schultz, T. Paul, and DaVanzo, Julie T.
  1970   Analysis of Demographic Change in East Pakistan: A Study of Retrospective Sur-
         vey Data. Publication no. R-564-AID. Santa Monica, Calif.: RAND.

CHAPTER 9

Relationships between Fertility and Mortality in Tropical Africa

P. Cantrelle
B. Ferry
J. Mondot

The relation between fertility and child mortality can be examined with data on aggregates or on individuals. Both approaches will be utilized in this chapter, although emphasis is placed on the latter source because of the well-known interpretive problems associated with the former. Because so few data are available with which to confront the question in tropical Africa, our results can only be considered suggestive.

AGGREGATE CROSS-SECTIONAL RELATIONS

Retrospective surveys, usually based on a sample of the population, have been conducted in many African countries since the 1950s. These provide the principal data for examining cross-sectional relations between mortality and fertility. Total fertility rates, infant mortality rates ($_1q_0$), second-year mortality rates ($_1q_1$), and rates of mortality in the first two years ($_2q_0$) have been computed by comparable methods for 12 countries by Coale (1966). The data are presented in Table 9.1. The zero-order correlation between total fertility and infant mortality rates among these countries is $-.38$. The correlation between total fertility and second-year death rates is $-.37$. The widely observed positive association between

TABLE 9.1

Fertility and Mortality in Twelve African Countries

Country	Year	Total Fertility Rate	Infant Mortality Rate $(_1q_0)$	Second-year mortality rate $(_1q_1)$
Dahomey	1961	6.4	.221	.077
Guinea	1954-1955	5.8	.246	.087
Upper Volta	1960-1961	6.5	.270	.096
Niger	1960	7.7	.211	.073
Angola	1940, 1950	5.8	.273	.098
Zaire	1955-1957	5.9	.163	.084
Cameroon	1960	4.9	.232	.082
Kenya	1962	6.8	.132	.043
Mozambique	1950	5.4	.212	.074
Rwanda	1952-1957	7.0	.156	.057
Tanzania	1957	6.4	.193	.066
Uganda	1956	6.7	.172	.058

Source: Coale, 1966.

these variables obviously does not prevail in tropical Africa, although the results are not statistically significant.

Within these 12 countries, the demographic rates have been computed for a total of 47 subregions. Data are presented in Table 9.2. Taking each of these regions as an observation, the correlation coefficient with total fertility rates is −.058 for infant mortality and −.061 for second-year mortality. Again, the relation is negative and statistically insignificant.

The absence of a strong positive relation is confirmed by analysis of data generated under different and somewhat more precise procedures. Table 9.3 presents figures for three regions in Senegal. Infant mortality rates vary by a factor of 4, whereas total fertility and general fertility rates show almost no variation. Urban Dakar has achieved a low infant mortality rate but no equivalent reduction in fertility. M. Francois (1973) has computed infant mortality in Gabon to be a high 229 per 1000 but total fertility to be a relatively low 4.2 children. Among the Foulani of Cameroon, the figures are 85 per 1000 and 3.5. Thus, every possible combination of levels of mortality and fertility is encountered in tropical Africa, and the overall pattern is one of little association between the two rates.

The absence of a demonstrable link between these two rates at the aggregate level apparently stems from the fact that intermediate variables, which act more directly upon these rates, are covering up the strong

TABLE 9.2

Fertility and Mortality of 47 Strata in Africa

Country	Year	Strata	Total fertility rate	Infant mortality rate ($_1q_0$)	Second-year mortality rate ($_2q_0$)
Dahomey	1961	North	6.1	.194	.248
		South	6.6	.232	.295
Guinea	1954-1955	Forest	5.7	.281	.353
		Fouta Djallcn	5.9	.228	.289
		Maritime	5.6	.238	.302
		Upper Guinea	6.1	.241	.306
Ivory Coast	1957-1958	First Secteur	7.3	.195	.249
Mali	1956-1958	Mopti	6.9	.344	.426
Niger	1960		7.7	.211	.269
Guinea Bissau	1950		4.8	.211	.269
Senegal	1957	Valley	6.3	.223	.283
Upper Volta	1960-1961	Mossi	6.7	.296	.371
		Peul	5.8	.195	.250
		Western	6.1	.241	.305
Angola	1940-1950	Benguela	6.8	.275	.346
		Bie	5.0	.228	.290
		Huila	5.4	.166	.213
		Luanda	6.4	.329	.409
		Malange	5.6	.276	.348
Central African Republic	1959	Central Oubangui	4.4	.212	.270
		Banda	4.1	.222	.282
		Mandjia	5.3	.210	.267
		Rivers	4.2	.183	.234

TABLE 9.2 (Continued)

Country	Year	Strata	Total fertility rate	Infant mortality rate ($1q_0$)	Second-year mortality rate ($2q_0$)
Zaire	1955–1957	Equator	5.0	.155	.199
		Katanga	8.2	.124	.159
		Kasal	5.9	.201	.286
		Kivu	7.1	.177	.226
		Kinshasa	6.7	.156	.200
		Eastern	4.0	.131	.167
North Cameroon	1960	Hills	5.8	.259	.327
		Moslems	3.5	.193	.246
		Plain	5.3	.246	.312
Berundi	1952–1957		6.4	.156	.204
Kenya	1962	Central	6.6	.098	.122
		Coast	5.4	.151	.193
		Eastern	6.8	.111	.140
		Nyanza	7.9	.193	.246
		Rift Valley	6.5	.089	.111
		Western	8.1	.170	.218
Mozambique	1950	Central	6.7	.254	.321
		North	5.0	.167	.214
		South	4.6	.201	.257
Rwanda	1952–1957		7.0	.156	.204
Tanzania	1957		6.4	.193	.246
Ugunda	1959	Buganda	5.4	.160	.205
		Eastern	6.1	.189	.242
		Northern	8.4	.174	.223
		Western	7.7	.161	.206

Source: Coale, 1966.

to work at the individual level and to consider the whole group of inter-mediate variables in order to examine the relationship. Unfortunately, data about these are rare in Africa as, indeed, in the other regions.

A systematic inventory of currently available quantitative knowledge relative to the intermediate variables is obviously highly desirable. As a first step, let us emphasize the importance of two of these: length of breastfeeding and postpartum amenorrhea, for which quantitative data are becoming available; and pathological factors, such as infection and nutrition.

PATHOLOGICAL FACTORS

Among factors separately or jointly determining child mortality and fertility are pathological factors. Their influence is particularly important in tropical Africa, where they form two specific groups: Infections and malnutrition.

With reference to their respective influence on childhood mortality and fertility, infections can be broken down into three categories:

1. Those with effect on mortality only, e.g., umbilical tetanus of the newborn child or measles after six months
2. Those with effect on fertility only, e.g., gonococcic diseases
3. Those with effect on both mortality and fertility, e.g., malaria, which is particularly serious when the child is about 1 year old, but which may also be responsible for miscarriages.

The importance of pathological factors is evidenced by Gabon, where high mortality conditions are accompanied by a high incidence of sterility from involuntary causes. We estimate that 25% of the women of reproductive age in Gabon suffer from primary sterility, to which secondary sterility should be added in order to gauge the total fertility effect. Pathological factors can account both for the high level of mortality and the low level of fertility in Gabon. A program of disease control will not necessarily re-duce fertility here; if anything, it should be expected to raise it. Health programs in tropical Africa have a potential for raising growth rates through both mortality declines and fertility increases. Our assessment is that on the whole control of infectious diseases in tropical Africa, without any change in other variables, would result in a rise in fertility. The influence of nutritional factors on fertility under current African conditions remains, in large part, in the realm of hypothesis.

TABLE 9.3

Fertility and Mortality Levels in Senegal

Site	Year	General fertility rate[a]	Total fertility rate[b]	Mortality per 1000 $1^q{}_0$	$1^q{}_1$
Rural					
Sine	1963-1965	217	6.8	238	182
	1963-1970	194	6.2	238	
Saloum	1963-1965	219	6.6	(130)[c]	125
Urban					
Dakar	1972	205	6.6	60	

Sources: Sine 1963-1965 and Saloum 1963-1965, Cantrelle (1969); Sine 1963-1970, Waltisperger (1974); Dakar, Ferry (1966).

[a]Annual births per 1000 women age 15-49.

[b]Average number of births that would occur to a woman surviving to the end of reproductive life under prevailing rates of childbearing.

[c]Probably underestimated.

LACTATION AND POSTPARTUM AMENORRHEA[1]

Breastfeeding in Africa

The importance of lactation should be particularly stressed since it has an influence on fertility and especially on childhood health and therefore on mortality. While the phenomenon may be easily measured, pediatricians, who are mainly concerned, have collected few data; the data reported here were obtained mainly from various economic papers, food surveys, and demographic studies.

It is extremely difficult accurately to determine the duration of lactation by countries and ethnic groups and even harder to establish trends. Out of more than 50 available documents covering 17 countries in North, West, Central, and East Africa between 1922 and 1974, 10 papers provide specific data on duration of lactation in terms of the child's age at weaning. Among the latter, 5 papers deal with surveys conducted on samples of

[1] This section draws extensively from a paper by Jacqueline M. Mondot-Bernard to be published by the OECD development center.

more than 400 children in northern Algeria (Tabutin, 1973), a rural area in
Senegal (Cantrelle, 1971), Ivory Coast (Bels, 1972), Zaire (Vis and Hennart, 1974), and Madagascar (INSRE, CINAM, INSEE, 1962).

Let us consider the period of breastfeeding, i.e., from the child's birth
to weaning, which is defined as the day breastfeeding stops or the point at
which the mother's milk will no longer form part of the child's food. The
period thus defined will indicate both breastfeeding exclusively and mixed
feeding, i.e., a regime including breastfeeding supplemented by animal
milk or other infant foods. Available survey data are presented in Table
9.4.

Although of uneven value, the data in Table 9.4 show that for Africa as a
whole there is a long average period of breastfeeding; it lasts between 12
and 36 months in extreme cases and is generally about 18–24 months.
However, in certain countries, such as Algeria, Ethiopia, Uganda,
Madagascar, and in large cities, the period is shorter, i.e., about 12
months.

Two cases, Algeria and Senegal, yield more precise indications of variations in the duration of breastfeeding. According to Tabutin (1973), the
mean duration of breastfeeding in Algeria is shorter in towns than in rural
areas (11.3 versus 14.4 months). This difference is probably underestimated because of the higher infant mortality in rural areas (14 versus
10.9% in 1968–1969.) He also finds that a larger number of women in
towns breastfeed their children less than 1 month or not at all (14.4% in
cities). Moreover, the mean duration of breastfeeding increases regularly
with the woman's age in both urban and rural areas. Because it is unlikely
that a woman's breastfeeding capacity changes significantly with age, this
finding suggests that younger generations have reduced the length of
breastfeeding. The process of intergenerational diffusion is slower in rural
areas, probably because of greater observance of traditional family customs and the unavailability of commercial weaning foods. Irrespective of
age, a literate woman breastfeeds much less than an illiterate one—7.5
months against 13.4 months overall average. With education held constant, mean duration of breastfeeding is higher in rural areas.

In Senegal, the mean period of breastfeeding in the rural area of Sine is
24.3 months (24.5 for boys and 24.1 for girls) (Cantrelle and Leridon,
1971). No significant differential was found according to birth order, which
suggests that the younger generations have retained ancestral customs.
According to the observations in Dakar (Ferry, 1975), the mean duration
of breastfeeding is 18.9 months, a substantially shorter period than that
found in Sine. A mean period of 18.9 months in Dakar cannot be interpreted as an indication that city mothers are averse to breastfeeding, but it
nevertheless evidences a progressive behavioral change in urban areas.

TABLE 9.4

Duration of Breastfeeding in Africa

Country	Number of children	Age at weaning (months)	Sources
Gambia			
Keneba remote village	44	18-24+	Thompson and Rahman (1967)
Rural area	69		Crapuchet and Paul-Pont (1967)
Guinea			
Rural		36+	Paulme (1954)
Ivory Coast			
Abidjan	97	13.5	Chapuis et al. (1967)
Rural		36-48	Adou (1967)
Cocody Town		12	Aye and Assi Adou (1966)
Abidjan illiterate women	900	12-24	Leroux (1972)
Katiola "Mangora" potters	280	Mode 12	Bels (1972)
		Mean 13	
Nigeria			
Lagos		12	Bassir (1957)
Rural		18-22	
Ibandan	380	14+	Matthews (1955)
Inesi rural	241	23.2	Martin et al. (1964)
Mali			
Dogon		24-36	Erny (1967)

TABLE 9.4 *(Continued)*

Country	Number of children	Age at weaning (months)	Sources
Senegal			
Khombole rural		16–24	Raquet (1956)
Wolof, sérère	69	19–36	Crapuchet and Paul-Pont (1967)
Fouta Toro Roucouleur		12–24	Wane (1969)
Dakar			
Wolof girls		24	Diop and Cross (1956)
Wolof boys		18	
Guinean peul		18	
Sine rural	8456	Mode 24	Cantrelle and Leviden (1971)
		Mean 24.3	
Dakar total	643	18.9	Ferry (1975)
Upper Volta			
Lobi region		24–30	Mazer (1961)
Burundi			
Suburb Bujumbura		18–30	Magos[a]
Cameroon			
Tingelin Fali		24	Malzy (1956)
Pahouins		18–24	Oto (1963)
Guiziga plain		24–36	Podlewski (1966)
Mountain Mofou		36	
Mountain Hina		24–36	
Congo			
Dolisie		18–24	Croce Spinelli (1967)

TABLE 9.4 (Continued)

Country	Number of children	Age at weaning (months)	Sources
Rwanda			
Usumbura-Bahutu		12+	Vincent (1954)
Babembe		18	
Astrida	100	Under 24	Duren[a]
Zaire			
Bambara rural		24-36	Mertens (1948)
Kasai	57	18-24	Brock and Autret (1952)
Kwango Basuku	500	15-19	Holemans et al. (1954)
Coquilhatville	100	12-24	Devreese[a]
Kinhasa			Lambillon[a]
Forest-lake			
Tumba	164	18-24	Vis and Hennart (1974)
Savana		24	
Highland tribes	400	18-36	
Ethiopia			
Soldier women	2000	12+	Huber and Ulm (1962)
Three villages			
1		12+	
2		12-	Knutsson and Mellbin (1969)
3		Early	
Kenya			
Masai		36	Brock and Autret (1952)
Uganda			
Baganda of Kampala	245	12-16	Welbourne (1963)
Baganda		12	Gerber and Dean (1964)

TABLE 9.4 *(Continued)*

Country	Number of children	Age at weaning (months)	Sources
Somalia			
Nomadic tribes			
North		18	Mousden (1950)
South		24	Lipparoni (1952)
Tanzania			
"Wahehe"		24	Moller (1961)
Wagago		36-48	
Wanyakynsa		24+	
Wachaga		24	
Bahaya		30-36	
Moshi		12-24	Sawaki et al. (1974)
Madagascar		Mode 7-12	Francois (1962)
		Mean 15	
Algeria (North)			
Urban	3187	11.3	Tabutin (1973)
Rural	6970	14.4	
Sudan			
South		24-36	Housden (1950)
North		Under 24	

aUnpublished data made available to authors.

Lactation and Fertility

Mean duration of breastfeeding can be related to two types of fertility indicators in the region: cumulative or completed fertility rates and birth intervals. As part of a sample survey on household consumption conducted in Madagascar in 1962, the duration of breastfeeding was assessed in 15 ethnic groups. The results can be compared with those of a sample fertility survey performed in 1966 (Table 9.5). No relationship between the mean age at weaning and the fertility rate appears in this case, but there is relatively little variation in the age at weaning. The relationship with birth intervals should provide a more precise indication of the effects of breastfeeding on fertility.

Data on lactation and fertility in Africa are scanty (Table 9.6) and hardly comparable, but they deserve some consideration: They concern Algeria, Senegal, Nigeria, Zaire, and Rwanda. Results across countries as well as within countries indicate that the later the average weaning age, the longer the average birth interval.

A more detailed study of the Sine region of Senegal (Cantrelle and Leridon, 1971) has shown that in the absence of mortality, the interval between live births is lengthened by 9 months when the weaning age is increased by one year within the weaning-age range of 12 to 36 months. This latter study also showed that the death of an infant, which is equivalent to weaning, has an impact on fertility. Similar events are described in several studies of historical demography. The results consistently show that death of an infant leads to a shorter interval between that birth and the next (Table 9.7). In his study on the Crulai population, Louis Henry considers all alternatives and concludes that the relation derives from the difference in the duration of breastfeeding, the child's death having interrupted the process.[2] This is a stochastic rather than a deterministic relationship, since all lactating women are not temporarily sterile, and the duration of postpartum amenorrhea and lactation is not the same for all women.

Breastfeeding and Postpartum Amenorrhea

The duration of postpartum amenorrhea in breastfeeding women has been compared with that of women who do not breastfeed because their children were stillborn or died within 5 days of birth. The few available studies (Table 9.8) show a mean duration of 60 days for nonbreastfeeding women. This period is almost identical in the populations considered, despite wide differences in environment.

[2] See also Chapter 2, by John Knodel, of this volume—Ed.

TABLE 9.5

Duration of Breastfeeding and Fertility in Madagascar

Area	Ethnic group	Mean age at weaning (in months)	General fertility rate (per 1000)	Total fertility rate	Completed fertility
Highlands	Merina	16)	220	7.7	5.4
	Sihanaka	11)	150	5.4	4.6
	Betsileo	15			
North	Tsimihéty	16	220	7.2	4.4
East	Berzanozano	17)			
	Betsimisaraka	12)	210	6.5	4.7
	Tanala	13)			
Southeast	Antaimoro	14)			
	Antefasy	13)	200	6.4	4.3
	Antaisaka	13)			
South	Bara	15)			
	Antadroy	11)	160	5.2	3.4
	Mahafaly	14)			
West	Sakalava	14)	210	6.7	3.4
	Makoa	13)			

Sources: Data on breastfeeding are from Francois (1962); and those on fertility from Francois, P. (unk.) and Gendreau (1966).

193

TABLE 9.6

Duration of Breastfeeding and Birth Intervals in Four African Countries

Country	Duration of breastfeeding (months)	Birth interval (months)	Number of cases observed
Algeria	11.9	25.4	About 8500 urban and rural women
1970	12.9	27.0	
Nigeria			
1955	23.2	35.5[a]	248 births
Senegal	0-11	25.1	
1963-1967	12-14	25.4	8456 births in the same
	21-23	32.5	region
	33-35	40.9	
Zaire			280
1958		26.5	Kinshasa[b] households
1960	27	34.7[a]	Bandibu
1960	27	27.9	Bashi[c]

Sources: Algerian data are from Republique Democratique Algerienne (1972); Nigerian data from Martin et al. (1964); Senegalese data from Cantrelle and Leridon (1971); and Zairian data from Romaniuk (1967).

[a]Sexual intercourse is prohibited for women during breastfeeding because the mothers know that there is no substitute for breast milk and that the baby is at risk if prolonged breastfeeding is denied to him.

[b]Data based on a survey made in 1960 by the bureau démographique, Kinshasa.

[c]Data from a survey made in 1960 by R. Deman; quoted in Romaniuk (1967).

For breastfeeding women (Table 9.9), the duration of postpartum amenorrhea is considerably lengthened, and, in general, the longer the period of breastfeeding, the longer the period of amenorrhea. However, the published data are not always accurate; moreover, they provide only averages, and the correlation should be based on individual data. For Dakar in Senegal, Table 9.10 shows the mean duration of amenorrhea with finer detail on the duration of breastfeeding. It can be seen that although amenorrhea responds monotonically to an increase in length of breastfeeding, the relation is somewhat irregular and possibly subject to diminishing returns. On average, an extension of breastfeeding produces an extension of postpartum amenorrhea that is about half as long.

In any case, it should be noted that breastfeeding lengthens birth intervals and, consequently, reduces fertility through physiological phenomena exemplified by postpartum amenorrhea.

TABLE 9.7

Birth Intervals according to Previous Child's Lifespan

	Previous child's lifespan			Sources
	0-5 months	6-11 months	12 months plus	
Le Mesnil				
i	20.6	26.4	27.2	Ganiage (1963)
n	176	229	710	
Canada, eighteenth century				
i	18.8	23.5	25	Henripin (1954)
n	482	65	545	
Tunis, nineteenth century				
i	18.4	23.2	27.5	Ganiage (1960)
n	125	42	670	
Mömmlingen, end of nineteenth century				
i	17.3	20.1	27.5	Knodel (1968)
n	72	62	1086	
Senegal: Sine, 1963-1967				
i	20.3	23.8	32.1	Cantrelle and Levidon (1971)
n	140	128	340	
Senegal: Dakar, 1972				
i	27.1	28.0	29.0	Ferry (forthcoming)
n	226	155	174	
Nigeria: Inesi village				
i		17.0[a]	35.5	Martin et al. (1964)
n		34	248	

Note: i denotes birth interval in months; n denotes number of cases.

[a]Total stillbirths and deaths under age of 1 year.

TABLE 9.8

Duration of Postpartum Amenorrhea among Nonbreastfeeding Women

Country and date	Number of cases	Mean duration of postpartum amenorrhea (days)	Sources
United States			
Baltimore (1934)	2285[a]		Peckman (1934)
Cincinnati (1940)	3946[a]		Stix (1970)
Spartanburg (1940)	2131[a]		
Boston (1966)	1712[b]	60	Salber (1966)
Britain			
Birmingham (1968)	93[b]	59	Cronin (1968)
France			
Cambrai (1969)	276[b]	58	Pascal (1969)
Asia and South America			
Bombay (1957)	30[b]	60	Basci (1957)
Chile (1965)	297[b]	60	Perez et al. (1971)
Taiwan (1966)	27[b]	48	Jain (1970)
Bangladesh (1969)		63	Lincoln Chen et al. (1970)
Africa			
Léopoldville (1960)		49	Lambillon[c]
Rwanda (1965)	50	60	Bonte and Van Balen (1915)[d]
Dakar, Senegal (1971)	35	43	Ferry (forthcoming)

[a]Number of births in figure represents total number of births in study (breastfed or not).
[b]Number of women.
[c]Lambillon, J., Unpublished information.
[d]Bonte and Van Balen (1915, pp. 97-100). Recalculated on the basis of 74% conception in the nine months after birth, using the Potter (1963) method (cycle without ovulation 2, average time to conceive on return of ovulation 5). 9 - 7 = 2 months. Time overestimated as no account taken of fetal loss.

TABLE 9.9

Duration of Postpartum Amenorrhea and Breastfeeding

Country and year	Number of cases	Duration (days) among breastfeeding women		Sources
		Amenorrhea	Breastfeeding	
India				
Mysore, Ramagaram villagers 1954		300–330		Tietze (1961)
Bombay, rural district 1959		390–450		
Bombay 1957	434	360	480	Basci (1957)
Taiwan				
1966	1208	270	390^a	Jain
1966	1636	336	468	
1966	2664	342	561	
1966	427	294	537^b	
Chile 1965	153	110	120	Perez et al. (1971)
Bangladesh 1969	83	510	300^c	Chen et al. (1974)
Somalia 1952	2957	570^d	660	Lipparoni (1952)
Nigeria 1955	380	400	600	Matthews (1955)

TABLE 9.9 (*Continued*)

Country and year	Number of cases	Duration (days) among breastfeeding women		Sources
		Amenorrhea	Breastfeeding	
Zaire Coquilhatville 1960	500	278	519	Devreese[f]
Rwanda Astrida 1960 1965	100 209	343 471[e]	360-540 540	Duren[f] Bonte and Van Balen (1965)
Ethiopia 1962	2000	405	365	Huber and Ulm (1962)
Senegal Dakar 1972	650	310	562	Ferry (forthcoming)
United States Baltimore 1934	2285	162	225	Peckham (1934)

[a]Insufficient lactation.
[b]Babies not yet weaned.
[c]Mean duration of complete breastfeeding as computed on the sample of 83 women from Chen(1974, Table 7, p. 289).
[d]Mean duration of amenorrhea is underestimated because for the women (62.5%) whose menstruation had resumed more than two years after birth, the exact moment of onset of menses is not known.
[e]Computed from data of Bonte and Van Balen (1965, Table 2).
[f]Unpublished information.

Several authors have investigated whether such temporary sterility of breastfeeding women varied according to certain characteristics. In the United States, Potter (1963) found, apart from breastfeeding, only a link with the mother's age. In Taiwan, Jain (1970) found no variations according to education or place of residence. But in India, Malkani and Mirchandani (1960) observed that postpartum amenorrhea was longer where per capita income was lower; they attributed this to a better nutritional level of people with higher incomes.

Is malnutrition responsible for the long periods of postpartum amenorrhea found in breastfeeding mothers in Africa? We have seen that there is no difference between the various samples of nonbreastfeeding women in Europe, Asia, and Africa. If malnutrition has an effect on the duration of amenorrhea, it appears to operate only when women breastfeed. But no data are available on the nutritional level of the women considered in the studies cited; comparable observations on the duration of amenorrhea and of breastfeeding as well as on the nutritional level of women would be needed in order to form an opinion.

CONCLUSION

It does not currently seem possible to assess the strength of mortality–fertility relations in Africa. The research conducted so far at a macrodemographic level does not establish conclusively the existence of a direct cause-and-effect relationship. In order to state the problem in adequate terms, it is essential to consider explicitly the intermediate variables through which the relationship must operate. Unfortunately, research conducted along these lines thus far has not led to a synthetic view; only a few of the intermediate variables involved in the relationship could be identified or studied.

Certainly data at the individual level are consistent with the presumption that there should be a positive relation between the two that is a product of the biological link through breastfeeding and postpartum amenorrhea. This relation should be fairly strong in Africa because surviving children are quite generally breastfed for long periods.

New specific research needs to be undertaken to supplement present knowledge of such variables and assess their relative weight in the relationship under consideration. Data from the world fertility survey or other surveys of reproductive histories, together with a sensibly designed typology of intervening variables, should permit better estimates of the potential effects of child mortality reductions on fertility in the region.

TABLE 9.10

Duration of Amenorrhea according to Duration of Breastfeeding,
Dakar, 1972

Duration of breastfeeding (months)	Duration of Amenorrhea (months)	Number of cases
No breastfeeding	1.45	35
1-8	4.5	13
9-14	5.8	57
15-20	10.7	386
21-26	13.4	137

Source: Ferry (forthcoming).

ACKNOWLEDGMENTS

We would like to thank Dr. Benoit for computational assistance.

REFERENCES

Aye, H. and J. Assi Adou
  1967 "Education sanitaire et sevrage en Côte d'Ivoire. In "Compte Rendu d'une Table Ronde sur le Sevrage en Afrique Noire. Premieres Journees Medicales d'Abidjan." Janvier.
Basci, P. J.
  1957 A natural history of child bearing in the hospital-class woman in Bombay. Journal of Obstetrics and Gynecology of India 8:26–51.
Bels, Anne
  1972 Fécondité, Mortalité de l'Enfance dans une Zone Rurale de la Côte d'Ivoire, Enquête Pilote chez les Potiéres Mangoro de Katiola.
Berman, M. L., Helman, and I. L. Hansonk
  1972 Effect of breastfeeding on postpartum menstruation, ovulation and pregnancy in Alaskan Eskimos. American Journal of Obstetrics and Gynecology 114(4):524–534.
Bonte, M. and H. Van Balen
  1965 Prolonged lactation and family spacing in Rwanda. Journal of Biosocial Science 1:97–100.
Brock, J. F. and M. Autret
  1952 Le Kwashiorkor en Afrique. Monographie No. 8. Geneve: World Health Organization.
Caldwell, J. C. (ed.)
  1973 "Introduction: Quelques questions importantes." Chapter 1 in Croissance Démographique et Evolution Socioéconomique en Afrique de l' Ouest. New York Population Council.

Cantrelle, P.
1969   "Etude démographique dans la région de Sine-Saloum (Sénégal)". Pp. 121 in Travaux et Documents, No. 1. Paris: ORSTOM.
Cantrelle, P. and H. Leridon.
1971   Breastfeeding, mortality in childhood, and fertility in a rural zone of Senegal. Population Studies (London):505–533.
Chapuis, Y., J. Assi Adou, and F. Paillerets
1967   "Pathologie du sevrage." Pp. 193–195 in "Compte Rendu d'une Table Ronde sur le Sevrage en Afrique Noire, Premieres Journees Medicales d'Abidjan." Janvier.
Charbonneau, Costallat
1954   L'allaitement maternel en milieu musulman; Enquete menée sur l'allaitement maternel à Fes. Maroc Medical 33:16–18.
Chen, et al.
1974   A prospective study of birth intervals in rural Bangladesh. Population Studies 28:277–297.
Coale, A. J.
1966   Estimates of fertility and mortality in tropical Africa. Population Index 32(2).
Crapuchet, S. and Ika Paul-Pont
1967   "Enquête sur les Conditions de Vie de l'Enfant en Milieu Rural au Sénégal et en Gambie." Pp. 3–25 in L'Enfant en Milieu Tropical, No. 39. Paris: Centre International de l'Enfance, Institut de Pédiatrie Sociale.
Croce Spinelli, Michel
1967   Les Enfants de Poto Poto. Paris: Grasset.
Cronin, T. J.
1968   Influence of lactation upon ovulation. Lancet (London) August.
Cros, J. and G. Senghor
1967   "Sevrage et éducation sanitaire." Pp. 197–201 in Compte Rendu d'une Table Ronde sur le Sevrage en Afarique Noire, Premieres Journees Medicales d'Abidjan. Janvier.
Day, R. L.
1967   Factors influencing offspring, number of children, interval between pregnancies and age of parents. American Journal of Diseases of Children 113(2):179–185.
Diop, S. and J. Cross
1956   "Aspects du Sevrage en Milieu Néo-urbain en Afrique." Pp. 56–57 in Conditions de Vie de L'Enfant en Milieu Urbain en Afrique. Paris: Centre International de l'Enfance.
Erny, Pierre
1967a   "L'allaitement dans la vie coutumière africaine." Pp. 40–44 in l'Enfant en Milieu Tropical, No. 39. Paris.
1967b   "L'Apprentissage de la Vie." Pp. 27–31 in l'Enfant en Milieu Tropical, No. 42. Paris.
Ferry, B.
1975   "Étude de la fécondité à Dakar (Sénégal). Principaux resultats d'ensemble." Bulletin de Liaison I.N.E.D., INSEE, ORSTOM, MICOOP. 18:40–47 (Octobre-Décembre). Paris.
1976   Etude de la Fécondité à Dakar (Sénégal). Ojectifs, Méthodologie et Résultats. Paris: ORSTOM, in press.
n.d.   Enquête sur la Fécondite à Dakar Paris: OSTROM. (forthcoming)
François, M.
1973   "Gabon." Pp. 854–888 in J. C. Caldwell (ed.), Croissance Démographique et Évolution Socio-Économique en Afrique de l'Ouest. New York Population Council.

Franņcois, P.
   unk.   "Allaitement et alimentation de sevrage des enfants. Budgets et alimentation des
          ménages ruraux en 1962 (Madagascar)." Pp. 63–66 in Nutrition et Sociologie
          Alimentaire, Vol. 2. Paris: INSRE/CINAM/INSEE.
Ganiage, Jean
   1960   La Population Européenne de Tunis au 19e Siecle. Paris: P.U.F.
   1963   "Trois village d'Ile-de-France. Etude démographique." Pp. 148 in Cahiers de
          Travaux et Documents, No. 40. Paris: INED.
Gautier, Etienne and Louis Henry
   1958   "La population de Crulai, paroisse normande. Etude historique." Pp. 272 in
          Cahiers de Travaux et Documents No. 33. Paris: INED.
Gendreau, F.
   1967   Enquête démographiqe, Madagascar 1966. Paris: ISRE.
Henripin, Jacques
   1954   "La population canadienne au debut du 18e siecle. Nuptialité, fécondité,
          mortalité." Pp. xxxii–118 in Cahiers de Travaux et Documents, No. 22. Paris:
          INED.
Henry, Louis
   1956   "Anciennes familles genevoises. Etude démographique: XVI–XX siecles." Pp. 234
          in Cahiers de Travaux et Documents, No. 26, Paris: INED.
Hiernaux, H. Vanderborght
   1956   "Croissance pondérale du nourrisson pendant la première année à Astrida." Bulle-
          tin de la Société Royale Belge d'Anthropologie et de Prehistoire 67:133–139.
Housden, Leslie
   1950   "Infant feeding in north-east Africa (notes based on experience in the Anglo-
          Egyption Sudan and Solaliland)." British Medical Journal (London) August: 456–
          457.
Huber A. and R. Ulm
   1962   "Probleme der Laktationsamenorrhoe (Untersuchungen in Aethiopien)."
          Gynaekologe (Berlin) 153:282–297.
Jain, A. K.
   1970   "Demographic aspects of lactation and post-partum amenorrhea." Demography
          7(2):255–271.
Jeliffe, D. B.
   1970   L'alimentation du nourrisson dans les régions tropicales et sub-tropicales (World
          Health Organization Monographie No. 29), 2nd edition. Geneve.
Knapen, M. T.
   1962   L'Enfant Mukongo. Orientations de Base du Système Educatif et Développemnt
          de la Personnalité. Louvain: Publications Universitaires.
Knodel, J.
   1968   "Infant mortality and fertility in three Bavarian villages: An analysis of family
          histories from the 19th century." Population Studies (London) 22(3):297–318.
Knutsson, K. E. and T. Mellbin
   1969   "Breastfeeding habits and cultural context (a study of three Ethiopian com-
          munities)." Journal of Tropical Pediatrics (London) 15(2):19–40.
Lacombe, B.
   1970   "Fakao Sénégal: Dépuoillement de registres paroissiaux et enquête démographique
          rétrospective." Pp. 156 in Travaux et Documents, No. 7. Paris: ORSTOM.
Leridon, H.
   1973   "Aspects biométriques de la fécondité humaine." Pp. xii–184 in Cahiers de
          Travaux et Document, No. 65. Paris: INED.

Leroux, S.
1973 "Ròle de l'équipe obstétricale dans la promotion de l'allaitement maternel dans la population." In Collogue sur l'Allaitement Maternel, Abidjan, 1H-16 Novembre. Paris: Centre International de l'Enfance.
Lipparoni, Egidio
1952 "Singolari aspetti dei cosi detti fenomeni simpatici della gravidanza, della funzione mammaria e della recomparsa del ciclo mestruale dopo il parto nelle donne somale." Archivio Italiano di Scienze Mediche Tropicali e di Parassitologia (Rome) 33(9):501–519.
Longo, L. D.
1964 "Socio-cultural practices relating to obstetrics and gynecology in a community of West Africa." American Journal of Obstetrics and Gynecology 89:470–475.
Malkani, P. K. and J. Mirchandani
1960 "Menstruation during lactation." Journal of Obstetrics and Gynecology of India (Bombay) 2:11–22.
Malzy, Pierre
1956 "Les Fali du Tingelin." Etudes Camerounaises, mars.
Martin, J. W., D. Morley, and M. Woodland
1964 "Intervals between births in a Nigerian village." Journal of Tropical Pediatrics (London) December: 83–85.
Matthews, D. S.
1955 "The ethnological and medical significance of breastfeeding with special reference to the Yorubas of Nigeria." Journal of Tropical Pediatrics (London) 1(1):9–24.
Mazer, André
1961 "Sevrage et mortalité infantile en pays Lobi (Haute-Volta)." Bulletin de l'Institut National d'Hygienne (Paris) 16(1):127–138.
Mertens, Victor
1948 "Le mariage chez les Mambara (Bakongo) et ses lecons sociales." Zaire 2(10).
Michaux, Didier
1972 "La démarche thérapeutique du NDOP, NDOP et sevrage." Psychopathologie Africaine (Dakar)   :17–57.
Moller, M. S. G.
1961 "Custom pregnancy and child rearing in Tanganika." Journal of Tropical Pediatrics (London) 7(2):66–80.
Nogue, Adam
1922 "La Mortinatalite et la mortalite infantile dans les colonies francaises." Pp. 5–29 in Congres de la Sante Publique et de la Prevoyance sociale, Marseille, 11–17 Septembre.
Ojiambo, J. A.
1967 "Background study of food habits of the Abasamia of Busia District, western province, Kenya." Nutrition (London) 27:216.
Omolulu, Adewale
1972 "Allaitement maternel au Nigeria." Pp. 19–24 in L'Enfant en Milieu Tropical, No. 82. Paris: Centre International de l'Enfrance, Institut de Pediatrie Sociale.
1974 "Importance de l'allaitement maternel." Afrique Medicale (Dakar), No. 120 (May):485.
Oto, I.
1963 Le Sevrage chez les Pahouins. Pp. 37–38 in L'Enfant en Milieu Tropical, No. 9. Paris: Centre International de l'Enfance, Institut de Pediatrie Sociale.
Pascal, Juliette (Soeur Marie-Christine)
1969 Quelques aspects de la physiologie du post-partum. Ph.D. thesis, Nancy, Faculté de Medecine.

Paulme, D.
    1954   Les Gens du riz. Paris: Plon.
Peckham, C. H.
    1934   "An investigation of some effects of pregnancy noted six weeks and one year after
           delivery." Johns Hopkins Hospital Bulletin 54:186–207.
Perez, A., P. Vela, R. Potter, and G. S. Masnick.
    1971   "Timing and sequence of resuming ovulation and menstruation after childbirth."
           Population Studies (London) 25(3):491–503.
Petros Barvazian, Angèle
    1975   Maternal and child health and breastfeeding. Milk and lactation. Modern problems
           in pediatrics. In S. Karger Basch (ed.), International Symposium on Milk and
           Lactation, Campione, September 9–12, 1973.
Podlewski, A. M.
    1966   La Dynamique des populations du Nord Cameroun. Serie Sciences Humaines, Vol.
           3, No. 4. Paris: ORSTOM.
    1970   "Un essai d'observation permanente des faits d'état-civil dans l'Adamaoua." Pp.
           150 in Travaux et Documents, No. 5. Paris: ORSTOM.
Potter, R. G.
    1963   "Birth intervals: Structure and change." Population Studies (London) 12:155–166.
Raquet, Jean
    1956   Contribution à l'étude du problème de l'allaitement maternel en Afrique (Sénégal)
           Ph.D. thesis, Dakar, Faculte de Medecine/Ed. Leconte.
Republique Democratique Algerienne
    1972   Résultats de l'enquête fécondité 1970. Alger, Novembre, Serie 2, Vol. 2, p. 111,
           143.
Republique de Senegal, Ministère des Finances, Direction de la Statistique
    unk.   Enquête Nationale Demographique: Methodologie et Documents Annexes. Dakar.
Romaniuk, Anatole
    1967   La Fécondité des Population Congolaises. Paris: Mouton.
Salber, Eva J.
    1956   "The effect of different feeding schedules on the growth of Bantu babies in the first
           week of life." Journal of Tropical Pediatrics (London) 2(2):97–102.
Salber, Eva J., M. Fedehleb, and B. MacMahon
    1966   "The duration of post-partum amenorrhea." American Journal of Epidemiology
           82:347–358.
Sanjur, Diva M., Joaquin Cravioto, Lydia Rosales, and André Van Veen
    1970   "Infant feeding and weaning practices in rural preindustrial setting: A socio-
           cultural approach." Acta Paediatrica Scandinavica (Stockholm), Supplement 200.
Sawaki, K., M. Zella, and M. Feyhold
    1974   "On the slopes of Kilimandjaro." Les Carnets de l'Enfance (Geneve) 28:2–16.
Senecal, J., G. Pille, Ch. Sayerse, and M. T. Ospital
    unk.   Examen du lait de femme africaine; mise au pointe de la technique. Medecine
           Infantile (Paris) 91–98.
Slome, Cecil
    1960   "Culture and the problem of human weaning." Journal of Tropical Pediatrics
           (London) 6:23–34.
Stix, R. K.
    1970   "Factors underlying individual and group differences in uncontrolled fertility."
           Milbank Memorial Fund Quarterly July 18:239–256.

Tabutin, Dominique
  1973   Quelques données sur l'allaitement en Algérie du Nord. Population (Paris) 6:1177–
         1186.
Thompson, B. and A. K. Rahman
  1967   "Infant feeding and child care in a west African village." Journal of Tropical
         Pediatrics (London) 3(3):124–138.
Tietze, Christopher
  1961   The effect of Breastfeeding on the Rate of Conception. Mimeograph prepared for
         the 1961 International Population Conference.
Vincent, Marc
  1954   "L'enfant au Rwanda Urandi." Institut Royal Colonial Belge 23(6):21–91.
Vis, Henri and Ph. Henmart
  1974   "L'allaitement maternel en Afrique centrale." Les Carnets de l'Enfance (Geneve)
         25:87–107.
Waltisperger, D.
  1974   Le Fichier de Population de N'Gayokheme (Sénégal). Analyse des Donnees 1963–
         1970. Dakar: ORSTOM.
Wane, Yaya
  1969   Les Toucouleurs de Fouta Toore, Sénégal. IFAN Bulletin (Dakar) 25. (Collection
         Initiations et Etudes Africaines).
Welbourne, H. F.
  1958   "Bottle feeding. A problem of modern civilization." Journal of tropical pediatrics
         (London) 3(4):157–165.
  1955   "The danger period during weaning. A study of Baganda children who were attend-
         ing child welfare clinics near Kampala, Uganda." Journal of tropical pediatrics
         (London) 1(1):34–46.
Wennen Van Dermey, C. A. M.
  1969   "Nigeria: Developing world. The decline of breastfeeding in Nigeria." Tropical and
         Geographical Medicine (Amsterdam) 21(1):93–96.

Part 3

ISSUES IN INTERPRETATION

CHAPTER 10

Measurement Problems in the Analysis of Linkages between Fertility and Child Mortality

W. Brass
J. C. Barrett

1. INTRODUCTION

Fertility and child mortality are related in many different ways. There is seldom any need to establish this. The relevant issue is the interpretation of the interactions. Understanding how the level of child mortality and changes in it may affect fertility requires identification of this particular form of relation in the presence of others. The purpose of this chapter is to outline the main problems of establishing the relevant effects and the possible methods of approach. It is intended to serve as a framework for discussion and not as a definitive study. With our present knowledge and stock of observations, it would be premature to attempt the latter.

2. CLASSIFICATION OF RELATIONS

A brief indication of the types of mortality–fertility relation which may exist is necessary to clarify the subsequent arguments. First, there are several ways in which statistical correlations can arise without any meaningful association. The most elementary are artifacts caused by the variability in the characteristics and the nature of the data collection. There are a number of "chance" factors which affect the size of families such as age at sterility of the woman. Since the probability of a child death varies with the length of exposure to risk and many other features such as the age of the mother and the parity of the birth, the chance variation is not neutral with respect to the relation of interest. As will be demonstrated later, these artificial interactions can operate in complex ways. Another kind of interference comes from heterogeneity of the population. For example, if both fertility and child mortality decrease with rising income, then there will be an association between the two characteristics which does not come from any influence of one on the other. From the present viewpoint, the relationship is irrelevant or spurious. A slightly different but similar effect is that of coincidence when time series are being compared; some factor or factors may cause systematic changes in both fertility and child mortality so that there is a positive or negative correlation between them. Of course, such nuisance effects through mediating variables are a difficulty in all studies of relations from observational data. There is no logical method of avoiding them, but the dangers in the present context are particularly great and methods for reducing or assessing their impact of primary importance.

The associations of direct determination may be in either direction. That the level of fertility can have an effect on child mortality is well established. Probabilities of survival are poorer for births to older women and women of higher parities; obviously these tend to occur in larger families. In abstract theoretical terms, this might be a reverse reflection of a making-up of births by couples whose children are subject to a high mortality, but there is a large weight of evidence that the more obvious explanation is the true one. To argue this fully would require a paper on its own, but it is here accepted as true. Thus in any analysis which shows a decrease in fertility with lowered child mortality, the possibility that the effect is from former to latter must be considered.

Within the category of influences, which are directed from the child mortality to fertility several subclasses need to be specified. The process may be volitional or nonvolitional. Of the latter kind, the most obvious and discussed example is the effect of an infant death on the postpartum infertility period of the mother. The expected waiting time until the resumption of fecundity is lessened, in whole or in part, through the reduced length of lactation. Other things being equal, the period of exposure to risk is shortened less for a child dying young than for one which survives. There is thus compensation acting through a biosocial mechanism and not through any consciously or unconsciously motivated activity. There are other possibilities for nonvolitional effects although less is known about these. Thus, if the nutritional level and health of the woman are factors in the age at menopause (there is some data to support the idea), early child deaths may reduce the burden on the mother and increase the total period of exposure to the risk of conception.

Volitional effects of child mortality on fertility are also conveniently subdivided into two classes which may be labelled family and community. In the former case, the deaths of children to a couple are a determining factor on the attempts to produce subsequent children. This may operate through the use of family planning when the desired number of surviving children (or an upper risk limit for that number) is achieved or through less closely controlled means such as frequency of intercourse and separations of husband and wife. Community effects come from a broad recognition by the couples in a population that the mean family size should be related to the average incidence of child mortality to meet the needs for survivors; in particular they imply that if child mortality falls fewer births are required. Although there is no certain link between family and community effects, it seems unlikely that the latter would occur without the former: The converse proposition is not so plausible. The separation of community and family components of variation is a difficult task for any demographic phenomena, and little progress has been made in the topic. To undertake the separation for the fertility–mortality relation would require a range and detail of data in addition to a sophistication of analysis at present beyond our resources. The problem will not be considered here.

The strategy for the detection and verification of the volitional influence of child mortality on fertility is easy to define if difficult to apply. First, those measures must be chosen which can plausibly be expected to display particular patterns if the volitional hypothesis is valid and which are insensitive to the influences of the other "nuisance" interactions; the possible quantitative biases from the latter must be assessed and eliminated where practicable. The strength of the case will increase with the variety and precision of the patterns postulated, since the possible interference of uncontrolled nuisance factors will then be less likely.

3. AGGREGATE STUDIES

In aggregate studies, the mortality and fertility measures analyzed are for groups of families. These are usually large groups, for example countries, regions, or districts, mainly because of the nature of the data available. There are, in fact, some possible advantages of large groups if these are culturally and socially homogeneous since the pattern of interaction may then be easier to discern, but smaller units in bigger numbers supply more repetition of similar basic measures in different conditions. The effects sought must be from the mixture of family and community factors which combine in the overall indices. The analysis may be cross-sectional, that is of aggregates at a given period, serial over time, or both. Commonly in cross-sectional studied, child mortality is one of a number of variables which are used to "explain" fertility by regression techniques. However, the possibility of interference from the sources described in section 2 is so great and the scope for eliminating these so small that the approach is not promising. The interpretation of time series for a single aggregate is only slightly less forbidding. There is an important extra advantage from the fact that the time dimension gives some guidance on the direction of the effects (changes in child mortality can be related to later fertility movements) but this is offset by the severe statistical problems of autocorrelation.

The investigation of time series for a number of aggregates which share the wider socioeconomic influences but with variations in impact and tempo is more attractive (for example regions or districts within a country). If there are good vital registration and adequate estimates of populations at risk, the choice of demographic measures is not critical. Child mortality is heavily concentrated in the first 3 years after birth. There is little gain in going beyond that interval in terms of extra numbers and considerable advantage in the concentration of the measure over a short age range for time specificity. The common division of mortality under 1 year from that in the second and third has little to recommend it in biological or social terms; if a separation is to be made, it would be better to separate of deaths under one month from the remainder. In practice, one index of mortality such as $_2q_0$, $_5q_0$ (probabilities of dying by 2 or 5 years) or $_5m_0$ (death rate in first 5 years) seems sufficient.

For fertility there is the important distinction between general and marital rates and the need to apply some kind of age standardization. There is good reason to believe that changes in marriage patterns are caused by factors different from those affecting family size, and it does not seem likely that child mortality is an influence on the former. The study then should be of age standardized marital fertility. The Princeton program on the European fertility transition used indirect standardization based on the rates of married Hutterites, but a variety of other approaches would be equally valid. In practice, the decisions are determined by the data available. The use of cruder measures, such as marital or general fertility, or even the crude birth rate, will not necessarily lead to serious distortions, compared with the uncontrolled variation, over periods when age and marriage patterns are altering little (for example in many historical studies).

A theoretical case can be made for the use of cohort rather than time-period measures. Clearly this is unimportant for early childhood mortality, but it might be speculated that any influence of this would operate through the subsequent actions of the cohorts of women who experienced a particular infant death incidence around their ages of greatest fertility. However, community effects could have a quite different time lag, and variability of response tempo would blur the sharpness of any impact. It seems unlikely that much is to be gained by the use of cohort methods at the present stage of knowledge, and the appropriate data are seldom available.

The general points above apply also when good registration statistics and population at risk estimates are not obtainable and substitute methods are required to derive the necessary measures. Further issues arise from the nature of the indirect techniques. Usually, the attempt will be to derive fertility and child mortality measures from data collected in censuses or large-scale demographic enquiries for subaggregates (districts for example). The only satisfactory source of information for the mortality estimates is of total children born and died to the younger women. There are reliable means for turning the proportion of children dead by age of mother into conventional indices, developed by Brass (see The Demography of Tropical Africa and elsewhere) and elaborated by Sullivan (1972) and Trussell (1975). These give convenient measures of child mortality for the present purpose; in particular an estimate of $_2q_0$ for the births in the few years previous to the enquiry is obtained from the reports on child deaths by women ages 20–24 years. The bias that exists because of the exclusion of higher parity births to older mothers may actually be an advantage here since the corresponding mortality can hardly have a family influence on fertility.

The derivation of an appropriate fertility index is not so straightforward. It may seem that the obvious measure is the mean completed family size of married women from the census or survey. But older women often understate the number of children born to them, and the error may vary in ways which distort the relations sought. Again, much of the childbearing of these women will have taken place *before* the period to which the child mortality applies. The use of estimates from population age distributions and stable models also has this latter disadvantage. In addition the results are critically dependent on the level of child mortality assumed, which may introduce serious biases into the analysis of the interactions. Reverse survival procedures are even more sensitive to the same problem. The technique for adjusting reported births in the previous year (or a recent period) to be consistent with the mean children born to the younger women is independent of the incidence of child deaths and gives a fertility level for about the same time as the mortality estimates. Where this method works, it is probably the most satisfactory for the present purpose, but it can be badly distorted by age reporting errors. (See for example The Demography of Tropical Africa). A decision on the best measurement must depend on particular circumstances. For example the "own child" version of reverse survivorship can give satisfactory values for very recent fertility if completeness of coverage and age reporting are good for young children. The measures are dependent on the child mortality estimates, but the effects of the resulting biases vary with the levels and differentials in the two sets of indices. They may not be critical. In practice, the final estimates of fertility levels are often arrived at after comparison and assessment of values found by different techniques. The averaging, time-diffuse nature of the operation is obviously a serious limitation in any attempt to relate secular trends in fertility to those of child mortality.

4. FAMILY STUDIES

In family studies, attempts are made to examine the relation between the deaths of children and the total numbers of births. This could, in theory, be done for couples, but the observations are more commonly taken from maternity histories of women. The specificity of the hypothesis and data give wider scope for the exclusion of nuisance factors in the interpretation of patterns, but the danger of artificial and irrelevant interactions is greater than for aggregates. Although there is an important practical distinction between prospective maternal history studies (where subsequent additional births are recorded after a base-line survey) and retrospective (where the records are entirely from statements about past events), the conceptual difference is small. If the existence and timing of events were reported accurately, the retrospective data could be put in a prospective form, apart from the women who disappeared from the population by death or migration. The latter effect is unlikely to be critical for the analysis of the mortality–fertility relations. Omissions and wrong timing of events (which may easily vary with family size and child deaths) are, however, a common feature of retrospective surveys and these could seriously hamper the search for significant results.

In the discussion of measurement problems, the development will be from the less to the more detailed investigations. Reference will be made to a program of computer simulation research into biases which is being undertaken by the authors. The basic simulation system of reproductive histories of women has been described and applied elsewhere. To it has been added provision for deaths of children at ages up to $1\frac{1}{2}$ years, with appropriate effects of deaths in any month on the distribution of the post-partum infertility period. Because birth spacing is one of the factors being studied, single child families were omitted. A brief outline of the simulation model is given in the appendix to this chapter. The investigation is at an early stage, and only the simpler simulations have so far been completed.

It is sufficiently obvious that no sound conclusions can be reached on the implications of the mortality–fertility correlations from a general sample of maternity histories without some control of the length of exposure to risk, since variations in this for individuals will dominate the associations. The most obvious way of doing this is by length of marriage (or union). This will not entirely remove the nuisance effects of heterogeneity of exposure, since women married at different ages will be included for periods of their lives over which fertility rates and the incidence of child mortality both vary. There is also the linked problem of sterility which may be associated with high child mortality and the numbers of children. In countries where age at marriage has a small variance, it seems likely that allowance for this factor would be very small; in these circumstances, control either through length of marriage or age should be adequate. However, this needs further investigation, as do the possible sterility interactions about which hardly anything is known. In these instances as in others, there is an advantage in keeping the age interval of child mortality short to avoid problems of biases in the exposure to the risk of death. The arguments for the aggregate situation also apply here.

For a fixed exposure to risk, the number of births per woman varies because of chance as well as systematic factors. The more children there are, the larger the numbers who would be expected to die, other things being equal. That the pattern is not a simple one is illustrated by the computer simulation results shown in Table 10.1 for women of completed fertility, married at age 20 years. Child mortality was kept constant for all birth orders and ages of mothers with .22 probability of dying by $1\frac{1}{2}$ years. The peculiar shape of the additional birth measures (that is excluding the child deaths) indicates that chance artifacts are operating.

It might seem intuitively more satisfactory to examine child mortality rates in relation to mean family sizes, but when this is done for the same simulation data, the outcome appears even more puzzling, as shown in Table 10.2. Here the mean births go down for families where the proportion of deaths is high although child mortality was kept constant in the model. A detailed examination shows that this is a chance artifact. In the conditions, a very high incidence of child deaths comes from chance variation about the expected value but this is more likely to happen when there is a small number of births than a large. An extremely low incidence

TABLE 10.1

Women of Completed Fertility Married at 20 Years, Constant Child
Mortality, Mean Births by Child Deaths

Child deaths	Number of women	Mean births	Additional births
0	430	5.91	5.91
1	750	7.61	6.61
2	685	9.16	7.16
3	502	10.46	7.46
4	254	11.13	7.13
5 and over	138	12.20	6.80

(for example zero) is also more likely to happen in small families, and this
accounts for the lower mean births in the group with mortality less than
25%. There are other possible biases, not built into this model, which
could be considered, but the chance artifact influences are clearly too
great for a direct attack through first order associations in the total data to
be promising.

The question remains whether the second-order features of the observations, that is the form of the joint distribution of child births and
deaths, can aid the interpretation of the relation. Analyses of this nature
have commonly been used in population genetics, for example to investigate family influences in spontaneous abortions. If a hypothesis that there
is a volitional effect of child mortality on fertility implies a different type of
distribution of deaths by births, appropriate tests may be developed. Approaches of this kind deserve study. In the computer simulation model
used for illustration, the distribution of the number of child deaths over
families of a fixed size is binomial. If there were a volitional mortality
influence, the variance of the distribution would be reduced; presumably

TABLE 10.2

Women of Completed Fertility Married at 20 Years, Constant Child
Mortality, Mean Births by Proportions of Children Dead

Child death rate	Number of women	Mean births
Less than 25%	1577	8.81
25% to less than 50%	1017	9.30
50% and over	165	5.82

the reduction would be absent or small for family sizes of two or three and become progressively larger with greater numbers of births. Although in observations there would be many more complications, because of the influences of fertility characteristics on child mortality (age of mother, order, spacing), as compared with the model, these might not be critical. Further gains could come from the examination of the distributional patterns for different lengths of exposure to risk, using data for cohorts of incomplete fertility at the time of the retrospective enquiry, since the volitional effects would be expected to have the biggest impact at the larger exposures.

When the births and child deaths to each woman can be arranged as a dated series of events in whole or in part, there are further analysis options. Such data are obtained from detailed maternity histories or prospective follow-up studies of subsequent births in a period to women whose previous birth and child death experience has been determined. It is now possible to eliminate the first order interference of chance correlations by relating child mortality up to some marker with subsequent fertility. This marker may be a fixed exposure to risk (as measured by length of marriage or, less satisfactorily, age) or an achieved family size, that is parity. In the former case, not all the chance association is removed. Thus families with the highest proportion of deaths for a fixed exposure will tend to be concentrated where the births are small in number; this may imply subfertility or even sterility.

For example, Table 10.3 shows, for the same model, the results of a prospective (or quasi-prospective) study, in which women married at age 20 are classified at age 30 by the mortality of their children and their subsequent births recorded. Here the chance concentration of low and high proportions of children dying in small families is reflected in the subsequent births through the correlation of reduced fertility in the first 10 years of marriage with the later experience. If number of births is taken as

TABLE 10.3

Women Aged 30 Married at 20 Years, Constant Child Mortality, Mean Subsequent Births by Proportions of Children Dead

Child death rate	Number of women	Mean subsequent births
Zero	1117	3.97
Over zero to less than 25%	520	5.04
25% to less than 50%	843	4.55
50% and over	327	3.92

the marker, so that comparisons are by subsequent fertility according to children surviving infancy for fixed parities, there are still possible biases through heterogeneity of the exposure to risk interval. For example, at lower parities there could be a tendency for the higher child mortalities to occur either to women marrying late or to those with short exposure intervals with highly concentrated births at the time of the enquiry; in either case, there would be a subsequent exposure to risk biased downwards. It would seem necessary, therefore, to make allowance for both exposure interval and parity in the analysis, although the former might be less critical. In particular, if the measurements studied were parity progression ratios, it might be sufficient to eliminate these women whose exposure following a birth of the relevant order was severely truncated.

With these reservations about some control of exposure, the most effective use of the data might be the calculation of the proportions of women with n children, r of whom died before some early age, who subsequently had additional births. If the enquiry were confined to women of completed fertility, the outcome would be a straightforward study of parity progression ratios, subdivided by previous child mortality. More commonly in developing countries, women of incomplete fertility would be included to improve the quality of the reporting and give more weight to events nearer in time; volitional effects might be suspected to be of recent origin. In these circumstances, the calculations would give measures which were composites over cohorts of a particular kind, depending on the distribution of women by exposure to the risk of childbearing and the degree of truncation of their subsequent recorded experience. Although the levels of the proportions proceeding to a further birth would have no absolute meaning, this is unimportant for the present purpose where it is the comparisons by fixed parity and varying child deaths that matter. The addition over cohorts could introduce biases in theory through trends in either fertility or child mortality. For example, falling incidences of death would mean, for a given parity, a smaller subsequent exposure to risk of fertility for women with low child mortality because these would be overweighted by the younger cohorts. Such biases, however, are likely to be very small and in general would not justify the more elaborate statistical methods which could be used to eliminate time-period trends.

Although the analysis procedure outlined would reduce the nuisance interference of some fertility–child mortality interactions, others remain. The most obvious are probably the nonvolitional, physiological, and social factors. Following a birth, there is a period within which the probability of a further conception is reduced; the size of the effect varies greatly among women and is strongly associated with the length of breastfeeding. In several studies of populations where children are breast-fed for 18 months or more, the average interval before full fecundity is effectively resumed has been about 11 months.

However, there are at least two inquiries that give delays of 18 months. There is some doubt whether this longer interval is a purely physiological phenomenon, perhaps attributable to poor maternal nutrition or social customs of reduced cohabitation of partners when the woman is lactating have also contributed. Whatever the exact causes, the evidence is over-whelming that when a child dies young the delay to the resumption of full fecundity is correspondingly less. If the death is in the first few weeks after birth, the average reduction in the postpartum infertility delay may be more than one year.

It is obvious that these interactions pose serious difficulties for the isolation of volitional effects whatever the method of analysis used. The particular concern here is with the parity progression approach. The higher the number of child deaths for a given parity, the greater the reduc-tion in average birth interval and also in the probability that the last child has failed to survive. The effective subsequent exposure to risk thus increases with the incidence of child deaths for a given parity. It may be speculated that such effects could be appreciable for short follow-up periods, that is in prospective type enquiries where women are asked about additions to their families after an interval, following the determina-tion of their demographic characteristics by a base-line survey. With long intervals, such as those automatically provided by surveys of cohorts of completed fertility the interference from this source may not be of great importance, particularly at lower parities. In all-cohort analyses, the situa-tion is still more complex, particularly when, as suggested, women with shorter intervals of exposure after the given parity are excluded.

The computer simulation model has been used to explore the possible sizes of the biases arising from post-partum infertility in parity and expo-sure controlled analyses. Table 10.4 shows a selection of results for cohorts of women of completed fertility, married at different ages. The mean births, following the child mortality experience of the first r born are shown.

Despite the substantial sampling fluctuations, it is clear that the mean subsequent births increase appreciably with the number of children dead for a fixed parity. The rise is of about one-third of a child for a movement from no deaths to the highest mortality groups for which there are suffi-cient numbers at risk for estimates to be reasonable. The model samples are not large enough for the variation to be specified in detail by parity and age at marriage of the women. In real populations of course, there would

TABLE 10.4

Women of Completed Fertility, Married at Different Ages, Constant Child Mortality, Mean Subsequent Births by Deaths in First r

Child deaths	3		4		5		6	
	Number of women	Mean subsequent births	Number of women	Mean subsequent births	Number of women	Mean subsequent births	Number of women	Mean subsequent births
Age 15 at marriage								
0	1350	7.99	996	7.14	778	6.39	570	5.64
1	1146	8.01	1172	7.16	1080	6.27	1000	5.49
2+	310	8.34	569	7.59	799	6.79	995	5.93
Age 20 at marriage								
0	1251	5.90	889	5.22	665	4.47	480	3.74
1	1092	6.06	1102	5.20	963	4.55	840	3.84
2+	341	6.20	584	5.45	808	4.65	961	3.96
Age 25 at marriage								
0	1198	4.12	854	3.43	586	2.83	393	2.21
1	933	4.24	928	3.57	823	2.88	675	2.32
2+	310	4.26	485	3.85	646	2.90	720	2.33

be other intervening factors not included here. It should be noted that these results are for post-partum infertility intervals which average about 11 months. Larger effects are, therefore, possible.

The introduction of a further control, on the period since marriage in which the r births took place, will allow for some part of this bias, namely, in the increase of the subsequent exposure to risk when children die but not necessarily the carryover effect of the postpartum infertility distribution following the last birth. This is the typical situation in a prospective survey. Further measures derived from the model reproductive histories are given in Table 10.5.

For short intervals of follow-up, there is a clear tendency for a lower proportion of women with no children dead to have a subsequent birth, but by the end of three years the difference has disappeared. Nor is there any evidence that the mean subsequent births are higher when the child mortality in the first r is more severe. The sample fluctuations are substantial, but the overall precision is sufficient to demonstrate that with the method of analysis the bias which comes from postpartum infertility is small if the follow-up interval is not too short or, presumably, if allowance is made for births where the postpartum effect may be carried over into the prospective period.

Although the more obvious reflections of variations in child mortality by fertility characteristics into the inverse relationship are removed by prospective or quasi-prospective forms of investigation, others without this property may be postulated. One possible mechanism is through birth spacing. There is evidence from developing countries that there can be heavy excess child mortality when births to a mother are closely concentrated. In several East African surveys of the 1950s, child mortality (both under 1 and under 5 years) was about twice as high when the mean birth interval was less than 3 years in comparison with the incidence for mothers with longer intervals. That such effects are far too large to be a consequence of the postpartum infertility interaction with child deaths is again illustrated by the computer simulation exercise.

Mean birth interval in years	Total births	Percentage of child mortality
Less than 3	21,511	22.3
3 and over	2,806	20.8

A more detailed breakdown of the data shows that the greater concentration of births because of child deaths has only an apparent effect of any consequence on the mortality for very low mean birth intervals; the pro-

TABLE 10.5

Women of Various Ages Married at 20 Years, Constant Child Mortality, Proportion Having Further Births by Time Intervals and Mean Subsequent Births by Deaths in First r

Age 25

Child deaths	1		2		3	
	0	1	0	1-2	0	1-3
Interval (years)						
1	53	57	44	52	22	31
2	74	77	77	80	67	75
3	83	83	91	93	87	90
5	88	87	96	96	96	97
Number of women	540	111	1083	493	220	290
Mean subsequent births	5.75	6.39	7.09	6.93	7.50	7.41

Age 30

Child deaths	3		4			5			6		
	0	1-3	0	1	2-4	0	1	2-5	0	1	2-6
Interval (years)											
1	37	37	41	43	54	41	41	51	31	35	41
2	62	56	68	72	79	70	75	75	69	73	76
3	70	66	79	84	89	86	89	86	86	88	86
5	77	72	87	90	91	95	94	92	91	93	94
Number of women	198	189	315	302	124	246	356	285	94	181	188
Mean subsequent births	3.31	3.10	4.26	4.52	4.42	5.07	4.83	4.70	5.12	5.12	5.16

TABLE 10.5 (Continued)

| | Age 35 | | | | | | | | | | | |
| | 5 | | | 6 | | | 7 | | | 8 | | |
Child deaths	0	1	2-5	0	1	2-6	0	1	2-7	0	1	2-8
Interval (years)												
1	25	19	29	30	28	36	37	34	37	41	35	34
2	43	42	40	52	43	55	66	60	64	65	62	66
3	50	47	48	61	53	66	78	72	72	83	79	81
5	58	54	51	70	65	71	85	79	82	91	87	88
Number of women	96	109	86	142	182	172	91	225	296	69	144	312
Mean subsequent births	1.46	1.41	1.45	2.15	1.99	2.13	2.68	2.61	2.72	3.36	2.97	2.98

portion of mothers thus affected is too small to introduce a significant bias with the broad classification shown. Equally, although in theory volitional effects of child deaths on subsequent births could contribute to the bias, they are unlikely to have more than a small influence. It should be noted that the observations show that the high child mortality with close birth spacing exists at short durations of marriage before volitional biases would be operative.

Accepting that there is a substantially higher child mortality with close birth spacing, the women experiencing these risks will tend to be those with high fecundity or consistently short postpartum infertility periods. Since these characteristics will presumably continue into the period of exposure to risk, subsequent to that for which the deaths for fixed parities are measured as a base, nuisance interactions are again a possibility. In this model, an effect which is from fertility to mortality will appear as the reverse in a parity progression type analysis, and it is far from clear how it could be eliminated.

There is some evidence to suggest that in high fertility populations the chance variation in birth intervals dominates the systematic fecundity and postpartum infertility components. If this is so, the source of bias discussed would be of limited nuisance value, but little is established with any certainty.

In order to investigate possible consequences of a relation between child mortality and birth spacing, modifications were made to the simulated model. The probability of the death of a child was made to depend on the number of births in the five years preceding his or her own birth increasing linearly with the concentration. Although this is a greatly simplified method of introducing a birth spacing influence on child mortality, it gives results which are in conformity with observations. It is consistent with the idea that the effect operates through the burden upon the mother of having several young children to rear at the same time. Among the simplifications made (through lack of knowledge to do otherwise) are the specification of relative effects on probabilities of dying as the same for each month of the first one and a half years, the disregard of the influences of births following each one simulated or of deaths of those born in the preceding five years, and the holding of child mortality at the standard level for the first five years of marriage. By trial, the change in child mortality with birth concentration was adjusted to give measures in accord with the East African evidence referred to previously. Table 10.6 indicates the variations in child mortality with parity and average spacing consequent on the model relations.

The measures in Table 10.7, showing the mean subsequent births by deaths in the first r, that is with control for parity, are parallel to those in

TABLE 10.6

Women of Completed Fertility Married at Age 20, Child Mortality Varies
With Birth Concentration, Mortality in First Year and a Half from Birth

Birth order	Probability of dying	Mean birth spacing (years)	Probability of dying
7 and less	.194	Zero to less than 2	.251
8 to 10	.201	2 to less than 2 1/2	.212
11 to 12	.220	2 1/2 and over	.177
13 and over	.236	Total	.211

Table 10.4. The addition of the birth concentration relation to child mortality increases the bias as would be expected. Although its size can not be estimated with any precision because of the sample errors, an increase from some half to two-thirds of a child in the mean subsequent births as mortality rises from zero to the highest levels is indicated. This is a substantial effect and it can not be claimed, plausibly, that the order of the maximum has been represented. A combination of a long postpartum infertility period and child mortality variations with birth concentration of the most extreme in the East African surveys would have raised the bias considerably.

The consequence of introducing the additional control of a fixed exposure to risk as well as parity before the examination of subsequent children born is investigated in Table 10.8. At first sight, the results may seem surprising. Despite the sampling errors there is a clear tendency for the mean subsequent births to decrease with the severer child mortality. On further consideration, the reason is apparent. Since child deaths increase the exposure to risk, women who, without such mortality, achieve the same parity in the same time as those so affected will tend to have a higher potential fertility, which is reflected in their later births. The exposure to risk differences are partly a result of the mortality relation with birth spacing and partly from postpartum infertility. The lack of any indication of a gradient on mean subsequent births in Table 10.5 where only the latter effect is present is probably due to compensating pressures. The exposure to risk is offset by the carryover of the postpartum infertility of the last birth into the prospective period.

The interaction just considered can be regarded as the consequence of population heterogeneity for factors (fecundity and length of postpartum infertility) which are associated with the measures whose relation is being investigated. It creates particular difficulties because the effects might be

TABLE 10.7

Women of Completed Fertility Married at Different Ages, Child Mortality Varies with Birth Concentration, Mean Subsequent Births by Deaths in First r

	3		4		5		6	
Child deaths	Number of women	Mean subsequent births	Number of women	Mean subsequent births	Number of women	Mean subsequent births	Number of women	Mean subsequent births
Age 20 at marriage								
0	1297	5.78	987	5.01	756	4.24	547	3.56
1	1070	6.24	1074	5.31	953	4.44	827	3.77
2+	321	6.26	522	5.66	751	4.92	902	4.21
Age 25 at marriage								
0	1191	4.11	869	3.32	588	2.76	396	2.22
1	981	4.28	945	3.61	851	2.93	698	2.34
2+	292	4.46	475	3.79	601	3.24	684	2.59

TABLE 10.8

Women of Specified Ages Married at 25 and 30 Years, Child Mortality Varies with Birth Concentration, Mean Subsequent Births by Deaths in First r

Risk exposure	1		2		3	
	20-25	25-30	20-25	25-30	20-25	25-30
Child deaths						
0	4.94	3.28	6.52	4.66	7.01	5.17
1+	4.04	3.40	6.54	4.39	7.15	5.07

Risk exposure	3		4		5		6	
	20-30	25-35	20-30	25-35	20-30	25-35	20-30	25-35
Child deaths								
0	3.48	1.96	4.55	2.93	4.89	3.28	5.29	3.76
1			4.42	2.86	5.05	3.31	4.94	3.52
2	3.04	1.59	4.64	2.57	4.75	3.11	5.16	3.77

present to a similar degree in all populations whereas other social and economic causes of heterogeneity will be less consistent. Nevertheless it should be realized that the latter type of bias is a danger in all attempts to establish causal relations from survey observations. The problems of defining the child mortality–fertility links are not more acute than comparable complications in other areas but rather among the more easily specified. Progress will come from an accumulation of consistent studies rather than one. There is great virtue in repetition in different conditions. Such repetition can sometimes usefully be achieved in single surveys by the analysis of relevant subsets of data, for example by culture or religion. It may also be illuminating to subdivide the observations according to indices of attitudes to child deaths and family sizes. If the indices have any validity, differences would be expected over the subdivisions in the measures designed to indicate volitional effects of mortality on fertility. The search is then for plausible patterns to confirm the relevance of the analytical approach.

APPENDIX

Model

In the Monte Carlo method adopted for this microanalytic simulation, events are represented individually; the parameters characterising natality and mortality are specified in the next section. This microanalytic approach permits greater realism, by allowing parameters to vary between women (or couples) and if necessary to depend on their ages, parities, or other desired factors, and facilitates the study of the relative effects of different parameters. The reproductive histories of a cohort of women are simulated from the beginning of marriage (usually at a fixed age) to the ends of the reproductive spans of life of the women (or couples), or until the woman's death. Events in this simulation occur only at intervals of one 'lunar' month, i.e., with 13 months to a year, which represents to sufficient accuracy the mean duration of a menstrual cycle. Commencing at marriage, there is a probability that a woman will conceive, equal to p per (lunar) month, which defines her fecundability. The fecundability p varies between women and declines with age as indicated in the next section. The history of each woman is simulated in turn through a series of states, the first of which is susceptibility to conception (i.e., the fecund state) and the second of which (if the woman is not by then sterile) is pregnancy leading to a fetal death (spontaneous abortion), stillbirth, or live birth. Induced abortions are not incorporated in the present work.

Although the simulation incorporates a family planning strategy (Barrett and Brass, 1974), this is not used in the present analysis.

Susceptible (Fecund) State

For this state, random numbers, Z, distributed uniformly between 0 and 1 are generated successively until a random number less than p (the fecundability to the particular woman) is obtained. In this way, a geometric distribution of times to conception is simulated, if p is constant, as it is taken to be until the woman reaches age 30. After age 30, fecundability starts to decline. Variation in fecundability between women is also incorporated: Values of p for women aged under 30 are drawn from a beta distribution

$$f(p) = p^{a-1} (1-p)^{b-1} / \int_0^1 x^{a-1} (1-x)^{b-1} dx$$

The parameters a and b were chosen to represent the distribution of completed family sizes in the population enumerated in the census of Ireland (1911), given the other components of the simulation. These components now include a decline in fecundability with age, which was not represented in an earlier version of the model (Barrett, 1971), so different values a and b are naturally required; these ($a = 3$, $b = 13$) turn out to be not very different from estimates made by Jain (1969) by a more direct method for Taiwanese women. To simulate the decline with age, the fecundability of a woman is redetermined at the beginning of each fecund interval, by linear interpolation, if she is over 30, between her original fecundability (as at age 30) and zero fecundability at her predetermined age of onset of sterility which varies between women. If she does not conceive within two years, her fecundability is redetermined in the same way and the process repeated until she conceives, becomes sterile, or dies.

Pregnant State

A further random number, Z, determines the outcome of pregnancy as a fetal death, stillbirth, or live birth, with probabilities θ_2, θ_3, θ_4 (where $\theta_2 + \theta_3 + \theta_4 = 1$). These probabilities are made to depend linearly on the woman's age, t years:

$$\theta_2 = 0.24 + [0.005 \, (t - 30)]$$

$$\theta_3 = 0.03 + [0.001 \, (t - 30)]$$

The duration of pregnancy is fixed for stillbirths and live births (9 and 10 lunar months) and is a geometrically distributed variate for fetal deaths. In the latter case, the proportion of fetal deaths that occur in the nth month is $.11\,(.55)^{n-2}$ for $2 \leqslant n \leqslant 8$; losses in the first month are discounted by the fecundability function. This representation is based on survey data analysed by French and Bierman (1952).

Insusceptible State

The interval of insusceptibility to conception, which follows the pregnant state, is taken as 2 months for a foetal death, 3 months for a stillbirth, and as a random variable with a Pascal distribution, following a live birth. The latter distribution is obtained as the sum of a constant delay of one month, followed by two consecutive goemetrically delays with parameters one-sixth per lunar month, giving a total mean delay of 11 lunar months, i.e., $1 + (1 - \gamma)/\gamma + (1 - \gamma)/\gamma$ where $\gamma = \frac{1}{6}$. These values are based mainly on surveys by Potter, Wyon, Parker, and Gordon (1965) and others. The advantages of a Pascal distribution in this connection have been discussed by Potter, Masnick, and Gendall (1973). In the present model, the first month following a live birth is supposed to be always anovalatory. The value $\gamma = \frac{1}{6}$ is modified when the child does not survive for $1\frac{1}{2}$ years, since the duration of lactation is affected. Thus if the infant dies at birth, $\gamma = \frac{1}{2}$, and the mean duration of the insusceptible state is then:

$$1 + \frac{1 - \gamma}{\gamma} + \frac{1 - \gamma}{\gamma} = 3 \text{ months.}$$

In general, when a child dies under $1\frac{1}{2}$ years, the *expected* duration of the interval of insusceptibility is interpolated between 3 and 11 months as follows. Let m be the (lunar) month of the child's age at death $(1 \leqslant m \leqslant 20)$. Define

$$h = \frac{4(m - 1)}{19} + 1$$

Then

$$\gamma = \frac{1}{1 + h} \qquad (\tfrac{1}{2} \geqslant r \geqslant \tfrac{1}{6}).$$

This representation is broadly in line with the regression of postpartum amenorrhea on lactation reported by Jain, Hsu, Freedman, and Chang (1970) and Jain and Sun (1972). There is thus considerable variability in the durations of the insusceptible intervals following live births even of children who die within $1\frac{1}{2}$ years. We note that in this respect the model differs from that of Ridley, Sheps, Lingner, and Menken (1967), who state, "In the computer program, if a child dies before the time selected at random for the duration of the post partum non-susceptible period, the non-susceptible state terminates one month after the infant's death" [p. 86]. The difference in the structures of these models seems to be of small importance for the present purpose, however, which is chiefly to estimate biases in mean values, and we have found that our estimates would not be much affected if instead the post partum period were truncated more sharply as indicated by Ridley *et al*. It may even happen, in the present model, that the death of a child actually appears to lengthen the duration of a hypothetical interval, since a new random variable is generated, but this is not to be regarded as a direct effect of the death. Instead, it represents a selection from the durations of insusceptible intervals of women of similar physiological status or experience following childbirth.

The parameters for the duration of the insusceptible interval do not vary between women here, the more important sources of heterogeneity having been provided in fecundability and sterility.

After each insusceptible interval in the present model, the woman returns to the suceptible state and conceives again, unless the end of the reproductive span is reached first, or unless she dies sooner. After each conception and each pregnancy, her age is tested to establish whether such an event has occurred, and if it has, the program causes summary statistics to be computed, before proceeding with the next woman's history, for up to, say, 3000 women.

Sterility

The sterility of a union, like fecundability, depends in reality on both the man and the woman, but for convenience of analysis is attributed entirely to the woman in the present model. It is represented as the lesser of two random variables. The first of these represents the woman's age at menopause, between ages 38 and 54, with mean 47.6 and mode 48.7:

$$f(\chi) = (\chi - 38)^2 (54 - \chi)K$$

The second random variable represents sterility occurring before menopause, at an age $28 + (Z/0.012)$, where Z is, as before, a random number distributed uniformly between 0 and 1. Also based on data for

Ireland (1911), 4.8% of women are deemed to be involuntarily sterile at ages under 28. The combination of these sterility effects gives a mean age of 43 and a median of 46 years at the end of the reproductive span (Barrett, 1971).

Child Mortality

For the present application, which is intended for developing countries, we use a fixed probability of .94 that the child survives the first month, followed by a conditional probability of .99 of surviving each month up to $1\frac{1}{2}$ years. The risk that the child dies is in the first instance taken as independent of the woman's age and parity, or rather it is not made to depend on these in the structure of the model, in order to find the separate direct effect of child mortality on fertility. But in subsequent runs, described in the text, the probabilities of dying (.06, .01) were multiplied by a factor $(s + 2)/4$ where s is the number of children born to the woman in the most recent 5 years, i.e., before the current birth. This represents a birth concentration effect on child mortality. It is thus possible for an involuntary effect to build up, by positive feedback, if the woman has a succession of births and deaths in a short interval.

Mortality of Women

The mortality of women (although not of their husbands) is represented here by means of the logit model of Brass (1972). It was needed for some current work on orphanhood and has little importance as regards the present investigation of biases. The logit $Y(x)$ of the proportion of females who survive from birth to age x is given by

$$Y(x) = \alpha + \beta \, Y_s(x)$$

where $Y_s(x)$ are the logits of the proportions surviving in the Brass standard population. The logit of a proportion p is defined as one-half the natural logarithm of $p/(1-p)$ and the α and β are parameters which generate sets of life tables from an initial pattern specified by the subscript s. In the present case, $\alpha = .022$ and $\beta = 1$, which implies that the mean expectation of life of female infants at birth is 44 years, and about 80% survive to their second birthday. The ages of the women at death are randomly selected from a life table formed from the values $Y(x)$, given that they all reach age 20.

All the random variates described in this appendix are generated independently of each other, insofar as sequences of pseudorandom numbers,

Z, are formed successively by multiplicative congruencies, i.e., from routines established for use with the CDC 6600 computer of the University of London.

REFERENCES

Barrett J. C.
1971   "Use of a fertility simulation model to refine measurement techniques." Demography 8, 481–490.
Barrett J. C. and W. Brass
1974   "Systematic and chance components in fertility measurement." Population Studies 28, 474–494.
Brass W.
1972   "On the scale of mortality." Pp. 69–110 in Biological Aspects of Demography. Taylor & Francis, Ltd.
French F. E. and J. M. Bierman
1952   "Probabilities of fetal mortality." Public Health Reports 67, 1161–67.
Jain A. K.
1969   "Fecundability and its relation to age in a sample of Taiwanese women." Population Studies 23, 69–85.
Jain A. K., T. C. Hsu, R. Freedman and M. C. Chang
1970   "Demographic aspects of lactation and postpartum amenorrhea." Demography 7(2), 255–69.
Jain A. K. and T. Sun
1972   "Inter-relationship between sociodemographic factors, lactation and postpartum amenorrhea." Demography India 1, 1–15.
Potter R. G., J. B., Wyon M. Parker and J. E. Gordon
1965   "A case study of birth interval dynamics" Population Studies 19, 81–96.
Potter R. G., G. S. Masnick and M. Gendall
1973   "Postamenorrheic versus postpartum strategies of contraception." Demography 10, 99–112.
Ridley J. C., M. C. Sheps J. W. Lingner and J. A. Menken
1967   "The effects of changing mortality on natality." Milbank Memorial Fund Quarterly 45 (1), 77–97.
Sullivan, J.,
1972   "Models for the estimation of the probability of dying between birth and exact ages of early childhood." Population Studies 26, 79–97.
Trussell, T. J.
1975   "A Re-estimation of the multiplying factors for the Brass technique for determining childhood survivorship rates." Population Studies 29, 97–107.

CHAPTER 11

Influence of Variations in Child Mortality on Fertility: A Simulation Model Study

K. Venkatacharya

The current unprecedented growth of population around the world has made it imperative to understand the causes of such growth. The two important factors that logically combine to produce it are fertility and mortality. In the recent past, many countries have shown significant declines in the level of mortality (United Nations, 1965). According to the theory of demographic transition, a slow decrease in fertility will gradually follow the decline in mortality as a result of economic, industrial, and urban growth (Blacker, 1947; Davis, 1949). Others suggest that reduced fertility is produced by the decline in mortality itself (Schultz, 1970). However, it has been argued that future declines in fertility in developing countries need not occur at the slow pace historically observed, in view of the many technological innovations in the control of human fertility. In this context, a study of the impact of declines of mortality in general and child mortality in particular on human fertility is of great interest.

OBJECTIVES

Mortality affects fertility and is in turn affected by it. Some of their interactions are direct and some indirect, involving a number of socioeconomic and cultural variables. Our attention will be focused only on measuring the impact of mortality on fertility. This impact can be studied to some extent through the analysis of historical data if such data are available and reasonably accurate. Studies using models can throw some light on the relationships, but the utility of the results depends to a large extent on the assumptions involved. The assumptions underlying models are dependent in turn on the amount of information or knowledge already available on the particular aspect under investigation. Thus, without enough data on the various intricate aspects of the problems under study, models, whatever their complexity, fail to add substantially to knowledge of the relations.

The present chapter is confined to analysis of the quantitative aspects of the impact of the decline in mortality on fertility. Its objective is to examine two problems connected with the direct and indirect effects of varying mortality levels in general and child mortality in particular on fertility. They are

1. How do various levels of mortality (including child mortality) and fertility result in different existing family sizes at different points of reproductive life?
2. Given parental preferences for a certain number or sex distribution of children, how does a family's history of child mortality and anticipation of subsequent mortality influence its size?

To answer these questions a cohort microsimulation model *(FERSIM)* using biological and demographic inputs has been developed. The model and the results are discussed later in the chapter.

REVIEW OF RELATED STUDIES

A decrease in the level of mortality can affect fertility in a number of ways. The increment in average marriage duration per couple as a result of decreasing mortality may have a significant effect on fertility by increasing the proportion married. In most of the developing countries where prolonged breastfeeding is quite common, a decrease in infant and early childhood mortality tends to increase the lactational period of mothers. Thus a decrease in mortality tends to increase both the length of lactational amenorrhea and the birth interval, resulting in lower average fertility per couple (Coale and Hoover, 1958; Hyrenius, 1958; Potter *et al.*, 1965; Ryder, 1955). Through the use of a computer simulation model, Ridley (1967) and her associates estimated that as $^0e_0$ (females) increased from 31 to 72 years, the live birth intervals increased by an average of 9 months for eighth order birth intervals, by 5 months for seventh order birth intervals and by 3 months for second order birth intervals under the specific assumptions and parametric values used in their model. The increase in mean birth interval of all orders was in the range of 5 months. The effect of lactational amenorrhea on fertility at different levels of mortality can be studied using steady-state results (Venkatacharya, 1974). As infant mortality decreases in the future, it will not necessarily be accompanied by an increase in lactation. The set of demographic variables that bring about declines in mortality (e.g., education of women) may tend to arrest increases in lactational duration or perhaps even to decrease it.

The indirect effect of declining mortality on fertility is more complex and less well understood. Knowledge of the changes in a couple's attitudes to fertility planning caused by declining infant and child mortality is essential for the formulation of any model, and this knowledge can be obtained only through carefully conducted field studies and surveys. A number of studies have shown that women's desires for additional births seem to be influenced to some extent by the number of their living children (Stycos, 1965:652; Gille and Pordoko, 1966:515, etc.). This is prima facie evidence that changes in mortality may induce changes in attitudes toward childbearing. A number of studies in developing countries have indicated that couples strongly desire to have at least one son alive during their old age (Operations Research Group, Baroda, 1973; Eliot, 1968; Hassan, 1967; Rizk, 1959). This preference for sons in India and other countries may result from a desire to carry on the family name and property, to receive economic and emotional support in old age, to assure the performance of religious rites, and to receive a helping hand on the farm and in the home. In countries like India, where there are no general old age social security schemes for the population, dependence on the son or sons in old age continues. Furthermore, in agriculturally based economies, a son becomes productive at an early age, despite laws forbidding child labor, thereby becoming an economic asset to the family. In a nationwide survey in India, 56% of couples wanted a son "to support family" and 42% "to carry on the line" (Operations Research Group, Baroda, 1973). Under such circumstances, the parents might plan their families in such a way that at least one son survives to old age.

Evidence of the effect of son preference on subsequent fertility of couples is not conclusive. One study in Taiwan found that the greater the number of sons the couple possesses, the lower the subsequent fertility (Heer and Wu, 1974). However, another study based on data from India, Bangladesh, and Morocco did not show any differentials in the subsequent fertility of couples with three male live births in comparison with those with three female live births (Repetto, 1972). A suggested explanation is that couples with one or more sons feel less "demographic pressure," as sons are less of a financial burden than daughters. Such families may feel the necessity of controlling fertility only toward the latter part of reproductive life and thus experience higher fertility.

High mortality combined with son preference is likely to influence subsequent fertility, especially if child loss occurs early in reproductive life. Some studies suggest that previous child loss impells couples to compensate for this loss (especially loss of a son) in their remaining reproductive life (Hassan, 1966; Wyon and Grodon, 1971; Harrington, 1971; Rutstein, 1970; Heer and Wu, 1974). However, one study did not show such a relation (Knodel, 1968). These studies suggest that the survival of a son, which in turn depends on child mortality, might influence the future fertility performance of a couple at any stage of their reproductive life.

The effect of sex preference in the presence of varying mortality levels has been explored extensively by Heer and his associates using simulation models (Heer and Smith, 1968, 1969; May and Heer, 1968). They have developed a model under the assumption "that parents have a perfect method of birth control but also want to be highly certain that at least one son will survive to the father's sixty-fifth birthday, so that he can support his parents in their old age." Heer and Smith's models brought out two important findings: *(a)* At the high mortality levels that are current in most of the developing countries, fairly large family sizes are required to insure the specified high survivorship of sons; *(b)* as the level of mortality fell from high death rate to low death rate, the impact on intrinsic rate of growth is curvilinear. When $^0e_0$ is less than 30, the improvements in mortality resulted in an increase in the intrinsic rate of growth, since mortality was still so high that birth control could rarely be implemented. When $^0e_0$ is 50, further improvements in mortality tend to decrease the intrinsic rate of growth, since an increasing number of women could stop childbearing at one or two sons in order to have at least a 95% chance of achieving one surviving son. One of the practical problems in applying the results of such models to real world situations is that most of the parents living in the rural parts of developing countries may have different mechanisms of insuring their son survivorship from one depending on their perceptions of son survivorship probabilities. Some of them might work with some simple rules, such as "three sons to be born to have one son surviving to old age." Survey material on the actual rules employed by parents is deficient. Furthermore, it is likely that parents might modify their son survivorship criteria as they proceed through life, as a result, for example, of changes in economic pressures on the family. The strength of motivation for surviving sons is also critical, and must be weighed against other family objectives such as minimizing immediate economic stress. The recent success of economic incentives in inducing mass sterilizations in India indicates that the motivation for son survivorship is probably neither rigid nor absolute.

A Monte Carlo simulation model has been developed by Immerwahr (1972) to study the variations in the chances that a father will be survived by his son(s) or daughter(s) under varying mortality, fertility, or both. If the level of Indian mortality in 1960–1961 had declined to that of the United States for whites in 1959–1961, the probability of a father being survived by at least one son would increase from .824 to .942, assuming in both cases that present Indian fertility prevails. If couples were to use a one-son limit, the corresponding probabilities would be .680 and .902. Immerwahr (1967) has also studied the probabilities of son survivorship under declining mortality and concluded that "the chances of a father being outlived by even one son are remarkably high, particularly after that son has lived the first two years of life."

THE MODEL

The model *(FERSIM)* used for the present work generates fertility histories of a cohort of women beginning with marriage and continuing until the age of 50 years or the dissolution of marriage, whichever happens first. Only first marriages are considered in the model (between ages 15 and 35 years) and marriage is assumed to be universal. The determination of events, such as marriage, is made by the usual method employed in Monte Carlo models. After marriage, the ages at death of the woman and the husband are determined. For this, the husband is assumed to be 5 years older than the wife, regardless of wife's age at marriage. The survival probabilities are those derived from the West model life tables (United Nations, 1967). The lowest value of the ages at death of the husband or the wife and the age of cessation of reproductive capacity, i.e., 50 years, is taken as the terminal age of procreation. Between the age of marriage and the terminal age of procreation, births are generated. The chance of giving birth is determined by probabilities corresponding to the monthly chance of conception; termination of a conception in a live birth, stillbirth, or abortion; termination of gestation; and the termination of postpartum amenorrhea following a live birth, stillbirth, or abortion. Once a birth occurs, the sex of the child is determined randomly using the sex-ratio at birth, assumed in the model to be 1.05 males per female. After the determination of the sex of the child, its age at death is determined. When the simulation of all births and related events for one married woman is com-

TABLE 11.1

Values of the Various Fertility Input Variables

1. Monthly chance of conception (MCC) by age in months (x),
    measured from month 169 (15 years old)

Level	x	MCC
F1	1 − 60	.05 + .0025x
	61 − 120	.20
	121 − 300	.20 − .00083(x − 120)
	301 − 419	.05 − .00042(x − 300)
F2	1 − 60	.03 + .0009166x
	61 − 120	.085
	121 − 180	.085 −.0005833(x − 120)
	181 − 240	.05 −.000466(x − 180)
	241 − 340	.0221 − .000201(x − 240)
	301 − 360	.01004 − 00015(x − 300)
	361 − 419	.001

2. Probability of conception termination in a live birth (L),
    stillbirth (S), or abortion (A) by 5-year age groups.

Age group	L	S	A
15−19	.806	.078	.116
20−24	.879	.048	.073
25−29	.895	.042	.063
30−34	.875	.050	.075
35−39	.829	.060	.103
40−49	.760	.090	.144

3. Mean value of the gestation period[a]

Outcome	Mean	Variance
Live birth	9.6 months	0.4
Stillbirth	8.1 months	0.6
Abortion	3.7 months	1.4

pleted, the same procedure is applied to the next woman. Histories of 600
women are simulated in three replicates of 200 women each. All output
tabulations are first made on the basis of 200 women, and later the results
are pooled. The size of 600 is sufficient for the analysis of most of the
output variables discussed in this chapter (Venkatacharya and Roy, 1972).

TABLE 11.1   *(Continued)*

---

4.   Mean value of the length of postpartum amenorrhea[a]

Outcome		Mean	Variance
Live birth	Level A1	17.4 months	24.29
	Level A2	10.59 months	38.70
Stillbirth		2.90 months	1.25
Abortion		1.50 months	0.45

5.   Mean age of marriage of a female[a]

	16.8 years	7.4

---

[a]In the simulation model, the various periods used are discrete probability distribution having these means and variances.

In the model, the level of mortality is assumed to remain constant for a period of 35 years, which is the maximum duration of marriage for any cohort. The model simulates fertility and mortality cohortwise and gives results for one generation.

Inputs

All probability density functions are discrete and numeric in form. In Table 11.1, only the mean values and variances of the probability distributions are presented. The distribution of age at marriage is based on Indian experience. Monthly chance of conception *(MCC)* is taken at two levels: The lower level is adapted from the estimates derived from the age-specific marital fertility rates of India (Venkatacharya and Roy, 1972); the higher level is chosen to correspond to a higher fertility pattern. The *MCC* is assumed to vary with the age of women only, but not with parity or between women, although the model *FERSIM* provides for both variations (Venkatacharya, 1971). The probability of a conception terminating in a live birth, stillbirth, or abortion is assumed to vary by 5-year age groups. The values of these probabilities are based on the Khanna study (Wyon and Gordon, 1971). The pregnancy periods leading to different types of outcome are based on Indian experience. The means and variances of these distributions are also shown in Table 11.1. The length of postpartum amenorrhea *(PPA)* takes on two levels. The lower level, with a mean of 10.4 months, is based on the Khanna study. The higher level, with a mean of 17.4 months, is chosen arbitrarily to reflect long breastfeeding. However, two runs (C9 and C10) are made to study separately the contribution of changes in lactation amenorrhea attributable to improving mortality. In the present paper, the length of lactational amenorrhea is kept constant under all levels of mortality except C9 and C10. In the model, primary sterility is ignored, but its effect can be taken care of by proper inflation of the results. Secondary sterility is not taken into account except through the lower monthly chance of conception assumed for later ages.

The other important input is the life table survival probabilities (p_x). The survival probabilities are available in the West model life tables by 5-year age groups. From these 5-year survival probabilities, single-year probabilities are obtained in two stages. For all ages above 5, the single year values are obtained by applying Sprague's multipliers to log (p_x), where p_xs are taken from West model life tables. For ages under 5, the single year figures are obtained by fitting a negative exponential curve to l_0, l_1, and l_5. In the model the mortality risk of each member of a family is assumed to be independent of others. Some of the characteristics of the life tables used in the model are shown in Table 11.2.

Output

Various types of fertility output are produced, including births by age of women, number of married women by age of the women, and single-year age-specific fertility rates; live birth intervals by 5 years of age and parity; number of children ever born and alive by sex for intact marriages of various durations; and the distribution of couples by number of sons and

TABLE 11.2

Some Indices of the Levels of Mortality (West model) Used

| | Level of mortality | | | | | |
	3	7	11	15	19	23
Males $(\overset{o}{e_o})$	22.85	32.48	42.12	51.83	61.23	71.19
Females $(\overset{o}{e_o})$	25.00	35.00	45.00	55.00	65.00	75.00
Life table infant mortality (1000 q_o) by level						
Males	351.3	248.2	171.7	111.4	62.9	21.4
Females	305.5	213.9	146.1	93.4	49.9	15.2
Life table childhood mortality (1000 $_4q_1$) by level						
Males	214.4	145.5	94.4	51.1	21.0	3.4
Females	215.5	145.6	93.7	50.5	19.0	2.4

daughters born. All of these outputs are obtained for each combination of input variables. The various combinations considered in this paper are shown in Table 11.3.

RESULTS

The input combinations C1, C2, and C3 provide three levels of fertility. While the input combination C3 generates fertility close to Indian experience, the other two patterns are arbitrarily chosen. The criterion used in their choice is that they yield an average of two and four live births more than C3 (for intact marriages by age 50 years). The mean number of births for intact marriages by age 50 under C3 is around six. In none of these simulations is fertility adjusted according to the number of living or ever-born children or sons.

Impact of Declining Mortality on Number of Living Children

Figure 11.1 illustrates the mean number of living children and living sons under six mortality levels (Table 11.2) for simulation C3. It indicates the extent of accumulated population pressure on families at various ages under different mortality regimes combined with the fertility regimes characteristic of India today. The mean values of the number of sons and children are obtained on women with intact marriages at that age. Thus, the mortality of the couples does not itself affect these values. The only difference between the various age trends shown in the figure is the mortality to which the children are exposed. It is clear that at low levels of mortality $[^0e_0(f) = 25,35]$, the mean number of living children increases linearly with age in the beginning, but actually declines at later ages. However, as mortality improves, the increase in the number of living children and living sons is monotonic. Similar results were obtained for simulations C2 and C1, although the level of surviving children is of course higher in these.

The percentage increase in the mean number of living children and sons for intact marriages by age 50 as mortality improves from level 11 $[^0e_0(f) = 45]$ to level 23 $[^0e_0(f) = 75]$ are shown in Table 11.4 for C1, C2, and C3. It is clear that when mortality improves, the percentage increase in the number of living children increases as fecundability decreases.[1] The reason is that as fecundability decreases in a pattern similar to that as-

---

[1] The same pattern would also apply to living sons if the sample of simulated women under each run were increased.

TABLE 11.3

Description of Input Combinations

Input combination	Monthly chance of conception	Postpartum amenorrhea	Son survivorship or other criteria
C1 (Medium fertility)	F1	A1)	None
C2 (High fertility)	F1	A2)	
C3 (Low fertility)	F2	A2)	
C4	F1	A1)	Fertility ends as soon as a son lives to 10 years.
C5	F1	A2)	
C6	F2	A2)	
C7	F1	A1)	Fertility ends as the presently born and the previous sons are alive, if the son born now is the second or third. For the fourth son born, fertility ends if the third and the fourth sons live another 5 years, otherwise the couple continues procreation until the end of reproductive life.
C8	F2	A2)	
C9	F1	A1)	No son survivorship criteria. Postpartum amenorrhea is assumed to depend on child survival.
C10	F2	A2)	

Note: All the combinations C1–C10 assume mortality to be constant with time. In all combinations C1–C8, *PPA* is assumed to be independent of child survival.

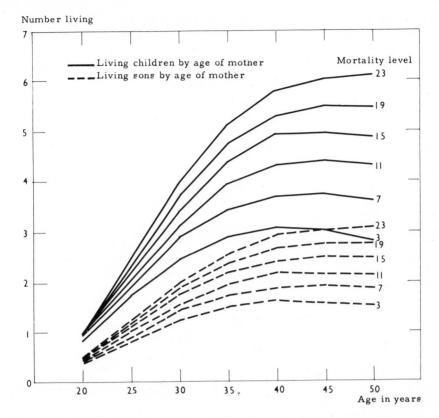

Figure 11.1. Number of living children and sons by age of mother, input combination C3.

TABLE 11.4

Effect of Mortality Improvement on Number of Living Children and Sons
for Women in Surviving Marriages at Age 50 under Three Different
Fertility Levels

	Mortality level (Coale-Demeny designation)				Percentage increase	
	11		23			
Simulation	Living sons	Living children	Living sons	Living children	Living sons	Living children
C2	3.53	7.39	5.22	10.21	48	38
C1	3.02	6.08	4.32	8.47	43	39
C3	2.09	4.26	3.02	6.03	45	42

sumed in this chapter, the proportion of male births or births occurring in the earlier reproductive years increases. Thus, the mean number of years a child has to survive from birth until the mother is aged 50 increases. Therefore, improvements in mortality have a slightly greater scope for influencing the mean number of living children at age 50 when fecundability is low than when it is high. Consequently, the proportionate effect of mortality change on the family's dependency burden is somewhat greater when fertility is low than when it is high, although the opposite is true for the absolute effect.

Impact on Fertility of Changes in Lactation Amenorrhea Brought about by Declining Mortality

In computer runs C9 and C10, the same input combinations are used as in C1 and C3, respectively, including the distribution of *PPA*. However, in C9 and C10 the *PPA* is made to depend on the survival of the child born. In these runs, a random *PPA* period is first selected, and this value is used if the child survives till the end of *PPA* of the mother. If the child dies earlier than the end of the selected *PPA,* the *PPA* is modified so that it is equal to 1 month more than the life of the dead child. Therefore, the results of C9 and C10 would be expected to be equal to C1 and C3, respectively, if every child survived to a period equal to the longest possible *PPA.* Thus, a comparison of the results of C1 and C3 with C9 and C10 indicates the impact of changes in *PPA* alone (under varying mortality levels) on fertility.

A study of age-specific marital fertility rates *(ASMFR)* obtained for the six mortality levels under C9 and C10 shows relatively small differences from the corresponding simulation C1 and C3. A comparison of the

TABLE 11.5

Age-specific Marital Fertility Rates (*ASMFR*) under Various Assumptions Regarding Effect of Child Death on Postpartum Amenorrhea

Age-group	ASMFR		Percentage increase	ASMFR		Percentage increase
	C1	C9		C3	C10	
15–19	.269	.296	10.1	.221	.245	10.9
20–24	.346	.357	3.2	.329	.335	1.8
25–29	.345	.347	0.6	.311	.316	1.6
30–34	.312	.312	2.8	.231	.234	1.5

[a]Higher ages are not shown because rates are based on fewer births, and stochastic error is correspondingly larger.

ASMFR (pooled for all six mortality levels) under C1 and C3 with the corresponding *ASMFR* under C9 and C10 is shown in Table 11.5, from which it is clear that the increase in *ASMFR* in C9 and C10 is small except for the first age group. The first age group shows a significant increase because most of the first births in that age group occur at 17–18 years of age (the last part of the age group), and the *PPA* following these births in C9 and C10 is on average shorter, leaving a greater chance for a woman to bear a second child in this interval than in C1 and C3.

The total number of live births for intact marriages by age 50 in C9 have increased by 3.1% from the corresponding values of C1 under mortality level 11. In the case of C10 the corresponding increase is found to be 2.5%. Thus, the effect on total fertility of linking lactational amenorrhea to child survival is hardly substantial. In C9 the mean number of live births is larger than the corresponding values of C1 for all levels of mortality, and the proportionate increase is much greater when mortality is high.

It would be expected that introducing a relationship between lactational amenorrhea and child survival would have a larger effect on fertility in a high mortality population. This expectation is confirmed in Table 11.6, which presents the cumulative fertility of women by age in simulations C1 and C9. A similar analysis made on the number of living children for intact marriages at various ages yielded analogous results.

Impact of Son Survivorship Criteria on Fertility under Improving Mortality

We shall now examine the impact of declining mortality on fertility as it operates through volitional mechanisms. As mentioned earlier in the

TABLE 11.6

Average Number of Children Ever Born to Women by Age under Four Combinations of Mortality and Fertility

| | Mortality level | | | | | |
| | 3 | | | 23 | | |
Age	C1	C9	Percentage increase	C1	C9	Percentage increase
25	2.64	2.83	7.3	2.74	2.77	.8
30	4.32	4.62	6.9	4.41	4.45	.8
35	5.93	6.24	5.2	5.97	6.04	1.3
40	7.19	7.63	6.2	7.28	7.38	1.3
45	8.23	8.61	4.6	8.28	8.33	.6
50	8.62	8.95	3.8	8.75	8.81	.7

chapter, little is known about how a couple assesses the level of mortality and how this level is functionally related to future fertility performance. We have made two different assumptions about the fertility motivation of parents. First, a couple is assumed to procreate until one son reaches the age of 10, at which point it terminates childbearing once and for all. Contraception is assumed to be perfect. The results under this assumption for the three patterns of fertility are labelled C4, C5, and C6, simulations that correspond in all other respects to C1, C2, and C3, respectively (Table 11.3). The second assumption is that a couple terminates procreation after the birth of a second or third son if a previous son is alive. If not, the couple continues to procreate, stopping only if, after the birth of a fourth son, both the third and fourth sons survive for five years. If on the other hand, one of them dies within five years (making a total of 3 son deaths out of 4 son births) the woman will not attempt to terminate fertility in her remaining reproductive life. Thus, the level of survival of recent births that is required to terminate reproduction is assumed to rise as child mortality in the family increases. Results under this assumption are shown

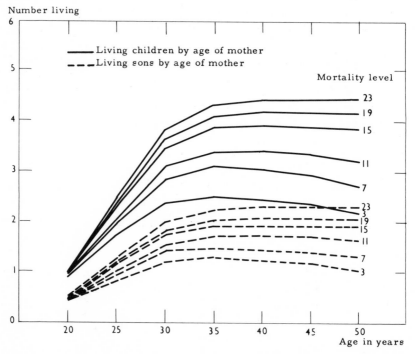

Figure 11.2. Number of living children and sons by age of mother, input combination C6.

for medium (C1) and low (C3) fertility patterns, and these are labelled C7 and C8, respectively.

Consider the results under the first assumption. Figure 11.2 illustrates the mean number of living children and sons at different ages of the mother in simulation C6. It is thus comparable to Figure 11.1, based on C3, except that a fertility-stopping rule has been added.

Although in all these runs it is assumed that fertility is terminated as soon as one son reaches the age of 10, the mean number of living sons by age 40 varies considerably. At mortality level three, the mean numbers of living sons are 1.25, 1.4, and 1.75 for C6, C4, and C5, respectively. This variation results from the fact that fertility is undisturbed for at least 10 years following the birth of a son. Higher fecundity populations continue to have larger family sizes.

The fact that fertility is inevitably undisturbed for a substantial period of married life also means that when mortality improves, the mean number of living sons and children increases despite the mortality-linked rule stopping childbearing. Table 11.7 shows that, whatever the level of fertility, the percentage increase in the mean number of living sons and children as a result of mortality improvement is substantial. The percentage increase in the mean number of living children increases as the fertility level decreases (C3 and C6), because more childbearing is concentrated in the early years of marriage in this simulation. Thus it is clear that the increased dependency burden brought about by improving mortality is large.

In Table 11.8, the *ASMFR* for C4, C5, and C6 are shown for each of the six mortality levels and compared to levels in C1, C2, and C3. In each of C4, C5, and C6, as mortality improves the *ASMFR* show a steady declining trend for ages above 30. For the younger groups, the trend is not

TABLE 11.7

Mean Number of Living Children and Sons of Women Aged 50 under Various Mortality and Fertility Regimes in Which Procreation is Assumed to Stop When One Son Reaches Age 10

| | Mortality level | | | | Percentage increase | |
| | 11 | | 23 | | | |
Simulation	Living sons	Living children	Living sons	Living children	Living sons	Living children
C4	1.978	3.709	2.411	4.840	22	31
C5	2.121	4.351	2.804	5.610	32	29
C6	1.654	3.186	2.261	4.428	37	39

TABLE 11.8

Age-specific Marital Fertility Rates (ASMFR) for Each Input Combination[a]

Input combination	Mortality level	Age group						
		15-19	20-24	25-29	30-34	35-39	40-44	45-49
C1[b]	All levels	269	346	345	312	217	184	93
C2[b]	All levels	307	427	426	384	308	206	102
C3[b]	All levels	221	329	311	231	135	54	8
C4	3	285	347	306	224	122	53	22
	7	300	346	312	191	93	33	12
	11	302	345	317	153	63	19	5
	15	300	350	300	161	62	18	3
	19	291	344	309	150	44	12	4
	23	296	358	295	122	31	7	1
C5	3	342	412	392	241	116	56	18
	7	331	426	382	203	87	27	7
	11	347	418	385	181	39	21	4
	15	330	435	394	175	53	11	5
	19	333	429	376	155	44	8	1
	23	324	421	373	153	35	10	2
C6	3	232	327	304	162	56	18	1
	7	250	335	289	144	51	16	2
	11	237	337	293	145	45	8	1
	15	230	346	301	130	32	8	1
	19	242	341	292	120	30	7	1
	23	232	340	296	115	26	5	0

TABLE 11.8 *(Continued)*

Input combination	Mortality level	Age group						
		15-19	20-24	25-29	30-34	35-39	40-44	45-49
C7	3	287	313	226	145	89	39	17
	7	293	306	219	126	67	30	14
	11	302	302	195	106	52	26	5
	15	296	296	176	84	33	15	5
	19	295	293	178	90	38	16	7
	23	287	289	175	73	28	12	3
C8	3	239	300	205	102	53	17	1
	7	233	313	196	101	44	13	3
	11	237	292	202	90	36	13	1
	15	231	305	184	88	32	9	1
	19	242	289	173	77	24	11	2
	23	237	286	171	71	28	5	3

[a]Input combinations are described in Table 11.3

[b]For these combinations, *ASMFR* does not vary by level of mortality. Thus, for each of these combinations all 6 x 600 case histories were used to obtain the rate. For each of the other combinations, only 600 cases were used.

TABLE 11.9

Intrinsic Growth Rate, Birth Rate, Death Rate, and Other Related Measures under Various Input Combinations (per 1000)

Input combinations	Mortality level	Growth rate	Birth rate	Death rate	Total fertility rate	Gross reproduction rate	Net reproduction rate
C1	3	15.86	66.72	50.86	8.41	4.10	1.57
	7	26.68	67.41	40.73	8.41	4.10	2.16
	11	34.14	66.95	32.81	8.41	4.10	2.70
	15	39.77	66.19	26.42	8.41	4.10	3.19
	19	44.07	65.35	21.29	8.41	4.10	3.66
	23	46.96	64.37	17.41	8.41	4.10	3.98
C4	3	8.70	53.81	45.08	6.36	3.10	1.26
	7	18.75	54.21	35.46	5.98	2.92	1.61
	11	24.90	52.69	27.80	5.56	2.78	1.86
	15	30.08	53.15	22.35	5.51	2.69	2.15
	19	34.48	52.07	17.60	5.33	2.60	2.34
	23	36.74	50.63	13.89	5.10	2.49	2.43
C2	3	22.96	80.64	57.68	10.31	5.03	1.93
	7	33.77	79.80	46.02	10.31	5.03	2.65
	11	41.22	78.22	37.00	10.31	5.03	3.31
	15	46.85	76.62	29.77	10.31	5.03	3.39
	19	51.14	75.19	24.04	10.31	5.03	4.46
	23	54.03	73.84	19.81	10.31	5.03	4.88
C5	3	14.91	64.94	50.03	7.36	3.59	1.47
	7	24.45	63.59	39.15	6.80	3.32	1.85
	11	31.43	62.69	31.26	6.45	3.14	2.16

TABLE 11.9 *(Continued)*

Input combinations	Mortality level	Growth rate	Birth rate	Death rate	Total fertility rate	Gross reproduction rate	Net reproduction rate
	15	37.92	63.47	25.54	6.50	3.17	2.54
	19	41.41	61.65	20.24	6.21	3.03	2.73
	23	43.80	60.10	16.30	6.09	2.97	2.90
C7	3	1.40	42.00	40.63	5.16	2.52	1.04
	7	11.00	42.49	31.49	4.84	2.36	1.32
	11	16.82	41.23	24.41	4.50	2.19	1.51
	15	19.89	38.48	18.59	4.10	2.00	1.61
	19	25.06	39.77	14.71	4.16	2.03	1.83
	23	26.31	37.42	11.11	3.92	1.91	1.87
C3	3	6.63	50.28	43.65	6.08	2.97	1.19
	7	17.90	52.87	34.96	6.08	2.97	1.62
	11	25.70	53.89	28.19	6.08	2.97	2.00
	15	31.63	54.32	22.70	6.08	2.97	2.35
	19	36.14	54.34	18.21	6.08	2.97	2.65
	23	39.18	53.88	14.70	6.08	2.97	2.89
C6	3	1.57	42.29	40.73	5.13	2.50	1.04
	7	12.77	45.04	32.27	5.03	2.46	1.37
	11	20.34	46.07	25.73	4.95	2.41	1.66
	15	26.16	46.68	20.52	4.87	2.38	1.91
	19	30.39	46.60	16.21	4.78	2.33	2.10
	23	32.97	45.71	12.74	4.70	2.29	2.24
C8	3	-5.94	32.04	37.98	4.21	2.06	.86
	7	5.37	34.94	29.56	4.15	2.03	1.14
	11	12.10	35.16	23.06	3.99	1.95	1.34
	15	17.49	35.53	18.04	3.89	1.90	1.52
	19	20.63	34.45	13.82	3.72	1.81	1.64
	23	23.08	33.65	10.57	3.64	1.78	1.73

decisive, largely because the reproductive stopping rule does not begin to affect behavior before the late 20s. Above this age, the probability of terminating fertility increases as the level of mortality improves.

It is important to compute the intrinsic rates implied by the various patterns of *ASMFR,* mortality. These rates are shown in Table 11.9. In each of simulations C4, C5, and C6, both the intrinsic growth rates and net reproduction rates increase as mortality improves, despite the fact that the total fertility rate and gross reproduction rate show a declining trend. The percentage increase in the net reproduction rate, as the level of mortality improves from level 11 to level 23, are 31, 34, and 35 for C4, C5, and C6. Fertility declines when mortality improves, but not by an amount sufficient to avert a major acceleration in growth.

Let us now turn to the second assumption. Figure 11.3 illustrates the number of living sons and children for women with intact marriages at different ages under simulation C8 (comparable to C3 and C6). The general remarks made with reference to C4–C6 hold in this case as well. When mortality improves from level 11 to level 23, the increase in the number of living children (for intact marriages by age 50) is 21.9% for C7 and 33.3% for C8. Once again, the percentage increase is larger for the lower fertility combination. Table 11.8 shows the *ASMFR* for C7 and C8. Except for the first age group, the *ASMFR* show a declining trend as mortality improves.

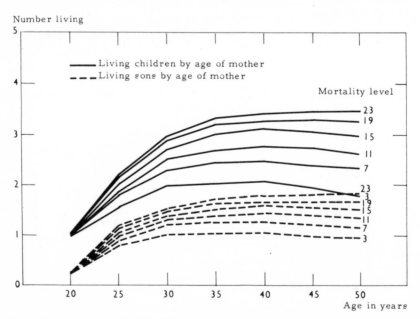

Figure 11.3. Number of living children and sons by age of mother, input combination C8.

Nevertheless, intrinsic growth rates and net reproduction rates rise markedly when mortality improves, as revealed in Table 11.9. The reduction in fertility by no means compensates for the reduction in mortality in its effects on growth.

In conclusion, this chapter shows that improvements in mortality tend to increase family dependency burdens, population growth rates, and net reproduction rates, even when families are assumed to employ a reproduction-stopping rule that is closely tied to the survivorship of previous births.

REFERENCES

Blacker, C. P.
  1947 "Stages in population growth." Eugenics Review 39:88–102.
Coale, A. J. and E. M. Hoover
  1958 Population Growth and Economic Development in Low Income Countries. New Jersey: Princeton University Press.
Davis, Kingsley
  1949 Human Society. New York: Macmillan.
Eliot, J. W.
  1968 Urban-Rural and Berber-Arab Differentials in Desired Numbers of Male Children and Related Factors in Algeria. Paper presented at the Annual Meeting of Population Association of America.
Gille, Halvor and R. H. Pardoko
  1966 "A family life study in East Java: Preliminary findings." Pp. 503–21 in Bernard Berelson et al. (eds.), Family Planning and Population Programs. Chicago: Chicago University Press.
Harrington, J.
  1971 "The effect of high infant and childhood mortality on fertility: The West African case." Concerned Demography 3:22–35.
Hassan, S. S.
  1966 Influence of Child Mortality on Fertility. Unpublished paper presented at the 1966 meeting of the Population Association of America.
  1967 Religion versus Child Mortality as a Cause of Differential Fertility. Paper presented at the annual meeting of the Population Association of America.
Heer, D. M. and D. O. Smith
  1968 "Mortality level, desired family size and population increase." Demography 5(1):104–21.
  1969 Mortality level, desired family size and population increase: Further variations in a basic model. Demography 6(2):141–49.
Heer, D. M. and Hsin-ying Wu
  1974 The effect of infant and child mortality and preference for sons upon fertility and family planning behaviour and attitudes in Taiwan. (Mimeograph.)
Hyrenius, H.
  1958 "Fertility and reproduction in a Swedish population group without family limitation." Population Studies 12:121–30.

Immerwahr, G. E.
1967 Survivorship of sons under conditions of improving mortality. Demography 4:710–20.
1972 Family Size and Survival—A Monte Carlo Model. Population Research by Computer Simulation. Project Report No. 15, International Institute for Population Studies, Bombay, India. (Mimeographed.)

Knodel, J.
1968 Infant mortality and fertility in three Bavarian villages: An analysis of family histories from the 19th century. Population Studies 22:297–318.

Knodel, J. and V. Prachuabmoh
1973 Desired family size in Thailand: Are responses meaningful? Demography 10(4):619–37.

May, D. A. and D. M. Heer
1968 Son survivorship motivation and family size in India: A computer simulation. Population Studies 22(2):199–210.

Operations Research Group, Baroda
1973 Family Planning Practices in India.

Potter, R. G., M. L. New, J. B. Wyon, and J. E. Gordon
1965 "Applications of field studies to research on the physiology of human reproduction. Pp. 143–173 in Mindel C. Sheps and Jeanne C. Ridley (eds.), Public Health and Population Change Current Research Issues. Pittsburg: University of Pittsburg Press.

Repetto, R.
1972 Son preference and fertility behaviour in developing countries. Studies in Family Planning 3(4):70–6.

Ridley, J. C., M. C. Sheps, J. W. Lingner and J. A. Menken
1967 The effects of changing mortality on natality: Some estimates from a simulation model. Milbank Memorial Fund Quarterly 45:77–97.

Rizk, Hanna
1959 Fertility Patterns in Selected Areas in Egypt. Unpublished Ph.D. Thesis, Princeton University.

Rutstein, S.
1970 "The relation of child mortality to fertility in Taiwan." Pp. 348–53 in 1970 Social Statistics Section, Proceedings of the American Statistical Association.

Ryder, N. B.
1955 "Influence of Declining Mortality on Swedish Reproductivity." Pp. 65–81 in Current Research in Human Fertility. New York: Milbank Memorial Fund.

Schultz, T. P.
1970 Analysis of Demographic Change in East Pakistan: A Study of Retrospective Survey Data. Rand Corporation.

Stycos, J. Mayone
1965 Social class and preferred family size in Peru. American Journal of Sociology 70:651–58.

United Nations
1965 Population Bulletin No. 7.
1967 Manual IV. Methods of Estimating Basic Demographic Measures from Incomplete Data. ST/SOA/Series A/42.
1968 The Concept of a Stable Population: Application to the Study of Populations of Countries with Incomplete Demographic Statistics. ST/SOA/Series A/39.

Venkatacharya, K.
1971 A Monte Carlo model for the study of human fertility under varying fecundability. Social Biology 18(4):406–15.
1972 Determination of sample size in the simulation models of human reproduction. Opsearch 9(1):19–29.
1974 A Comparison of Simulated Results with Those Obtained by Steady Stae Formulae. Proceedings of the Seminar on Computational Statistics, Vienna.
Venkatacharya, K. and T. K. Roy
1972 Estimation of monthly chance of conception from age specific marital fertility rates. Sankhya. B.
Wyon, J. B. and J. Gordon
1971 The Khanna study: Population problems in rural Punjab. Cambridge: Harvard University Press.

Index

Statistical difficulties in establishing
  associations, *see* Biases in measured
  relations
Sterility, *see also* Fertility control, 13, 183
Stopping probabilities, as influenced by
  child mortality in Israel, 169–172, *see
  also* Parity progression ratios
Sweden, 55, 56

T

Taiwan, 2, 94–98, 106, 139–152, 158
Time series relations between mortality and
  fertility, 179
  difficulties of interpretation, 210

in Europe, 50–57, 62–67
preferred methods of studying, 211–215

U

Uganda, 187

V

Volitional effects, *see* Replacement
  response; Extrafamilial effects

Z

Zaire, 192